Law and Nursing

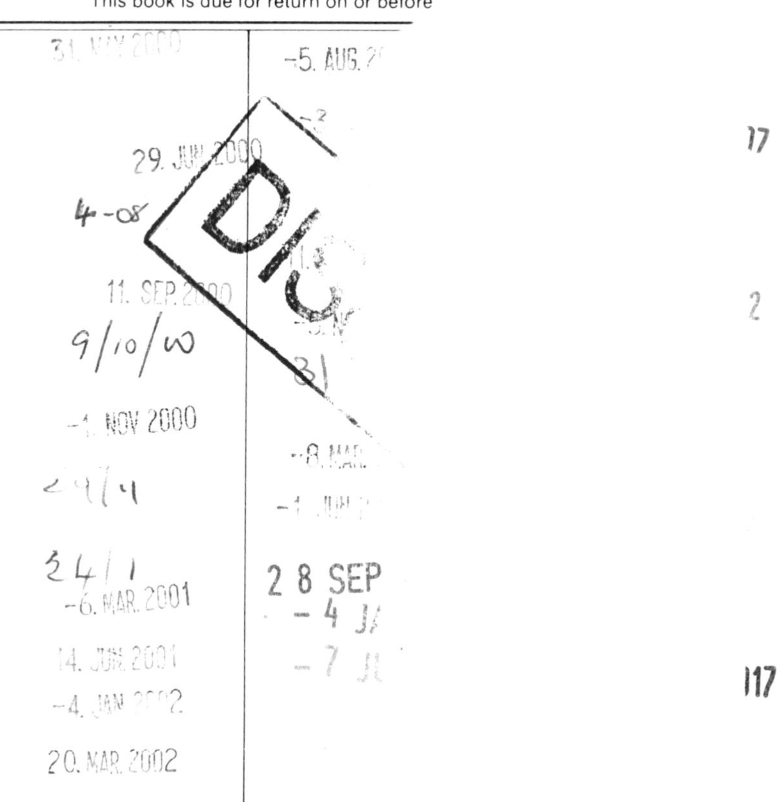

Errata

In Appendices 2 and 3, extracts are reproduced with kind permission of HMSO from '*Complaints Listening, Acting, Improving*' *Guidance on the Implementation of the NHS Complaints Procedure*, March 1996, NHSE. Diagrams are based on those contained in that booklet.

On page 184, paragraph 2, second sentence should read:
'In such a situation, the midwife should inform the mother of the legal position and that while she may refuse qualified help, an unqualified person who assists her may be prosecuted.'

On page 185, last paragraph, second sentence, the words 'While a woman is liable to prosecution should she refuse the assistance of a midwife' should be deleted.

Law and Nursing

Jean McHale LLB, MPhil
Lecturer, Faculty of Law, University of Manchester;
Director, Centre for Social Ethics and Policy,
University of Manchester, UK

John Tingle BA, Cert Ed, MEd
Barrister; Reader in Health Law; Director of the Centre for
Health Law, Nottingham Law School, The Nottingham Trent
University, UK; Visiting Professor of Law, Loyola University,
Chicago, USA

John Peysner MA
Solicitor; Principal Research Fellow, Nottingham Law
School, The Nottingham Trent University, UK

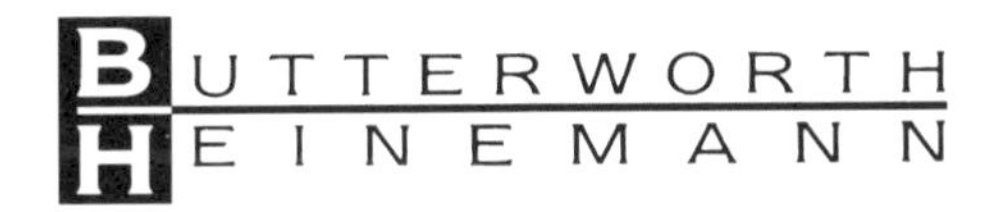

Butterworth-Heinemann
Linacre House, Jordan Hill, Oxford OX2 8DP
A division of Reed Educational and Professional Publishing Ltd

A member of the Reed Elsevier plc group

OXFORD BOSTON JOHANNESBURG
MELBOURNE NEW DELHI SINGAPORE

First published 1998

British Library Cataloguing in Publication Data
A catalogue record for this book is available from the British Library

Library of Congress Cataloguing in Publication Data
A catalogue record for this book is available from the Library of Congress

ISBN 0 7506 1594 X

Composition by Scribe Design, Gillingham, Kent
Printed and bound in Great Britain by
Biddles Ltd, Guildford and King's Lynn

Contents

Preface

The law and its relationship with nursing practice has increased in scope and complexity in recent years. Rarely a day goes past without a health care issue being in the headlines for one reason or another, whether in the form of National Health Service reorganisation, the prosecution of a health care professional or a decision to withdraw treatment from an incompetent patient. Legal issues are now featuring prominently on the nursing syllabus and are also of importance to many nurses undergoing further and postgraduate education. We hope that this book is not only timely, but that it will provide the nurse with an accessible and reasonably comprehensive guide to her or his legal obligations. The book is not intended to be a substitute for specialist legal advice on specific problems which may arise in individual cases. In addition, as this field is so vast in some areas, the account provided must be seen as a 'taster' for further, more extensive reading of specialist legal sources.

In the text reference is made to a wide range of decisions of the courts in decided cases. Cases are reported in the Law Reports of which there are various series. Some report a wide range of cases such as the All England Law reports and the Official series Law Reports such as the Queens Bench Reports (QBD) or Appeal Cases (AC). Some are specialist reports for example, the Family Law Reports which report cases concerning family matters such as treatment decisions involving child patients or Industrial Relations Law Reports (IRLR). Reference is also made to a wide range of literature published by the National Health Service Executive in Leeds such as Executive letters (EL).

Nursing law is an area increasingly affected by developments in Europe, some of which are considered in this book. An example of this, too late to be incorporated at proof-stage, which may have an impact on health care practice is the Council of Europe draft *Convention on Human Rights and Biomedicine.*

This book could not have been written without the help and support of a large number of people. Particular thanks go to Caroline Bridge,

William Bingley, Theresa Burgoyne, John Dybll, Carol Hall, Nina Fletcher, Marie Fox, John Hodgson, Maggie Mallik, Lynne McLachan, Vanessa Myatt and John Murphy, who discussed points with us and read through drafts at an earlier stage. All comments expressed and errors which remain are, of course, the responsibility of the authors.

Very special thanks go to the editorial team at Butterworth-Heinemann and, in particular, to Susan Devlin for her immense patience, kindness and encouragement through the long writing process.

The law is as stated on 1 January 1997. Since this date there have been a number of notable developments. At proof-stage a few amendments were possible to take on board the Nurses, Midwives and Health Visitors Act 1997.

Jean McHale
John Tingle
John Peysner

Case list

Numbers in **bold** are page numbers in this book.

Cases

AC	Law Reports, Appeal Cases
AJLR	Australian Law Journal Reports
All ER	All England Law Reports
BMLR	Butterworths Medico-Legal Reports
CMLR	Common Market Law Reports
CR App R	Criminal Appeal Reports
Crim LR	Criminal Law Review
DLR	Dominion Law Reports
EHRR	European Human Rights Reports
Fam Law	Family Division Law Reports
FLR	Family Law Reports
ICR	Industrial Cases Reports
KB	Law Reports, King's Bench
Med LR	Medical Law Reports
QB	Law Reports, Queen's Bench Division
SC	Session Cases
SLT	Scots Law Times
Sol J	Solicitors Journal
WLR	Weekly Law Reports

Australian cases:

Canadian cases:

USA cases:

European cases:

Health Service Commissioner decisions

Statutes and statutory instruments

SI	**Statutory Instrument**
NHSME EL	**National Health Service Management Executive, Executive Letter**

Acts of Parliament:

International Treaties and Declarations:

Secondary Legislation: SIs, Orders and Regulations

Miscellaneous:

Chapter 1

Introduction: The nurse and the legal environment

Jean McHale

In recent years legal issues in relation to the nurse's role have never been far from the headlines: 'Nurse performs operation'; 'Nurse blows the whistle on poor standards of care'. Many nurses have expressed concern regarding their legal obligations at a time in which the structure of health care provision is subject to almost constant change. At the same time the role of the nurse has evolved. Today, nurses perform tasks which would in the past have been undertaken by doctors. Nurses are also being encouraged to act as advocate for their patients, to safeguard standards of care and to speak out where those standards may be at risk.

The legal environment affects nurses in many ways, from the law of negligence concerning breaches of the legal duty of care to patients and others, to the nursing professions' governing body, the United Kingdom Central Council for Nursing, Midwifery and Health Visiting (UKCC), which is established under statute (Nurses, Midwives and Health Visitors Act 1997). In recent years the courts have been faced with many issues relating to health care practice, from the decision to withdraw treatment from patients in persistent vegetative state, to consent to treatment from negligence actions brought when patients have suffered harm during operations, to prosecutions where mercy killings have taken place. The structure of health care provision has been affected by legislation, most notably the introduction of the National Health Service (NHS) 'internal market' in 1991; the pace of change of law in this area and of professional practice has been rapid. Notable recent developments considered in this book include the new NHS complaints procedure and the recommendations regarding medical malpractice litigation proposed by Lord Woolf in his recent report (Woolf, 1996). There has been an increase in the number of negligence actions brought against health care practitioners. The scope of liability in negligence is considered below. Accompanying this has been the development of risk management practices aimed at reducing the prospect of litigation.

The evolution of nursing practice with the development of expanded role have led to concerns that the nurse should not be placed in a position where s/he may be called upon to undertake tasks which go beyond the scope of professional competence. The UKCC (1992) has issued a document, *Scope of Professional Practice*, which addresses many of these issues. The issue of expanded role is discussed further in Chapter 4.

This book attempts to provide nurses with an account of their legal obligations, whether studying Law as part of diploma or degree courses, or as a busy practitioner seeking clarification of her or his legal position. This is a book on nursing law written by lawyers for nurses. Although many ethical issues do arise in relation to the health care law matters in this book, the ethical debate is not addressed specifically; for that the reader is referred to the many health care ethics texts available (e.g. Tingle and Cribb, 1995). While it illustrates some of the legal dilemmas which arise, this book should not be seen as a substitute for the need to obtain specialist legal advice if particular problems occur.

This introductory chapter considers the framework of law and regulation within which the nurse practices. First, the structure of the English legal system and the nature of law, legal proceedings and court system are considered, then the structure of the NHS and finally the role of the nurse in relation to her or his professional body. The professional obligations of the nurse have been affected by recent guidance upon the scope of the nurse's professional practice. This guidance is considered in detail in this book and reproduced in the appendices.

Law and the legal system

Types of law

The legal system is divided into two main branches: criminal and civil law. **Criminal law** is a system for the state punishment of offences. In a criminal law case the action is usually brought by the Crown against the defendant. An individual may bring a private prosecution, but in practice these are very rare. A criminal law case is referred to as *Regina* versus *Smith*, which means the Crown against Smith or, as it is usually written, *R* v. *Smith*.

Civil law is the term given to an action brought by a person who has suffered some harm or loss - known as the plaintiff - against another person or organisation - the defendant. A civil law case is normally referred to as *Bloggs* v. *Smith*. The types of civil law action with which the nurse is most likely to be concerned are claims for breach of contract and actions in 'tort'. A tort is a civil wrong. Examples of torts include undertaking surgery without obtaining any form of consent from the patient (a battery), and failing to monitor oxygen levels during an operation with the patient as a consequence suffering brain damage (negligence). Other civil law actions include the action for breach of confidence in which the plaintiff claims that there has been unauthorised disclosure of confidential information entrusted to another in confidence. In civil law actions the plaintiff seeks a remedy usually in the form of financial compensation – damages. In addition, s/he may claim an 'injunction' to stop a particular type of conduct. An injunction is an order stopping the party performing the unjustified act. A contract is a legally enforceable promise, enforceable because both parties have given something of value. Examples include contracts of employment and contracts for sale of goods.

Public law

In some situations a person may want to challenge a decision of a Government body, health authority or other public body. S/he may claim that the body went beyond powers given to it by statute or that it has wrongly exercised a discretion granted under statute. Claims against public bodies in such situations should usually be brought through a special procedure known as 'judicial review'. Judicial review is not an appeal; the court cannot substitute its own view as to how the public authority should have behaved. Instead, the court determines whether the public body has acted legally.

A number of special remedies are available against public authorities through judicial review. An action can be brought seeking a 'declaration' from the court - asking the court to declare the law on a specific point. So for example, in *Gillick* v. *West Norfolk and Wisbech AHA*, Mrs Victoria Gillick went to court to ask for a declaration as to whether guidance given to health authorities that doctors could give contraceptive advice and treatment to girls under 16 years of age without parental consent was lawful ([1986] 1 AC 112). There are a number of what are known as 'prerogative writs'. One prerogative writ is the order of 'certiorari', which is obtained to quash an improper decision. The court may issue an order of 'mandamus' to require a public body to undertake its statutory duties. Perhaps the most well known prerogative writ is that of 'habeas corpus' in criminal cases, which is the requirement that the defendant be released from custody and the 'body' delivered to the applicant.

Types of court

Criminal courts

The magistrates court is a local court. Magistrates try minor criminal offences. In addition they hear evidence in relation to more serious criminal offences before committing these cases for trial at the Crown Court. In the Crown Court cases are heard by a judge, usually sitting with a jury of 12 lay persons selected at random from persons drawn from the electoral register in the local community.

Civil courts

The court in which a civil law case is heard usually depends upon the amount of damages claimed which relates to the degree of harm caused. Claims under £50 000 are usually heard in the County Court; claims over that figure are heard in the High Court. In civil cases the hearing is usually before a judge. Use of juries in civil cases is very rare today, the most notable example being libel cases.

Specialist courts/tribunals

In addition to the two main categories of courts outlined above there are also a number of specialist courts dealing with issues such as family law, or in the case of coroners' courts examinations into unexplained deaths. Hundreds of different bodies known as tribunals hear matters ranging from unfair dismissal claims in the context of industrial tribunals to immigration appeals. A tribunal chairperson is normally legally qualified. For instance, in industrial tribunals the chairperson usually sits to decide the case along with two other persons; one person is drawn from employers' organisations and the other from trade union organisations. Tribunals are less formal than the courts, with more flexible procedures in relation to calling witnesses and hearing evidence. There is also no automatic right to legal representation or to legal aid.

The upper courts

High court

There are three divisions of the High Court: the Chancery and Family Divisions hear exclusively civil law matters; and the Queen's Bench Division hears criminal law and public law matters. Each division is headed by a senior judge: in the case of the Chancery Division, the Vice-Chancellor, in the case of the Family Division, the President and the Lord Chief Justice for the Queen's Bench Division. These judges also sit in the Court of Appeal. The High Court may hear cases taken on appeal from the lower courts. Alternatively, cases may be heard for the first time in the High Courts. As noted above, such cases would include serious negligence cases.

Court of Appeal

Above the High Court is the Court of Appeal. This is composed of senior judges known as Lord Justices of Appeal. It hears appeals in both civil and criminal cases. The civil division is headed by the Master of the Rolls, the criminal division by the Lord Chief Justice.

House of Lords

The highest court within the United Kingdom is the House of Lords. It is composed of senior judges known as Law Lords. The Lord Chancellor presides over the House of Lords. He is a political appointment and also is a member of the Cabinet. This court bears the same name as the second chamber of Parliament, the House of Lords. Peers who have a right to sit in the House of Lords do not have the right to sit as judges in the court, but the Law Lords may participate in parliamentary debates.

Access to justice

One of the main restrictions upon use of the court process is that of the cost involved in bringing a case. There is a system of state funded legal advice, assistance and representation known as legal aid ((s1) Legal Aid Act 1988). Generally, applicants seeking legal aid are subject to a means test of their income and disposable capital to determine their eligibility. Much criticism has been levied at the fact that the threshold for disposable income and capital above which you are not entitled to free legal aid is very low. In a situation in which a person's income and disposable capital are higher than the levels of eligibility, then s/he may be required to make contributions in accordance with income levels. At present less than 50% of households are eligible for legal aid, and cuts in funding are continuing to reduce this figure (at one point some 80% qualified). Many cases, however, will be funded by legal expense insurance, for example individuals involved in road accident cases, and trade union members have access to legal support.

Alternative methods of funding of legal services have been suggested. One option is for the American model of 'contingency fee' to be adopted. That system operates by a lawyer taking on a client's case without requiring the client to make any initial financial contribution to the legal fees, but if the client's case succeeds, the lawyer then takes an agreed percentage of any damages recovered. In this country what are known as 'conditional fees for civil law cases' have been introduced (s58 Courts and Legal Services Act 1990). These allow lawyers to take on cases without the client incurring any cost for representation, but instead of allowing a percentage claim, the lawyer can recover a higher fee offset against the damages awarded in a successful action. Conditional fees are available for accident cases and they are backed by insurance; payment of a modest premium covers the person bringing the claim against any cost if s/he loses. At present, this insurance scheme is not generally available for medical negligence cases.

Settlements

While a dispute may lead to parties seeking legal advice and beginning legal proceedings, that does not mean that a case will ultimately go to court. Frequently, cases are settled before proceedings in court have begun. Indeed the threat of legal proceedings may operate as a negotiating tool, encouraging parties to settle their differences.

Sources of law

There are a number of sources of law. First, Acts of Parliament (also known as statutes), second, case law (derived from cases decided in the courts of law). In addition, English law is in some cases governed by laws laid down in Europe because we are parties to the European Union (see p. 9). A number of rules considered below govern how we assess what source of law contains the appropriate legal ruling in a situation.

Statutes

English law is to be found in Acts of Parliament. There are many Acts of Parliament relevant to nursing practice such as the Human Fertilisation and Embryology Act 1990 regulating infertility treatment, or the Abortion Act 1967. In addition, the nurse is affected by those statutes that apply more generally to the population as a whole, such as the Health and Safety at Work Act 1974. Statutes are being continually passed to govern new problems as they arise. A new statute may repeal an earlier statute, or it may amend it either in whole or in part. Statutes may also codify a particular area of law which was previously to be found in a large number of cases, or consolidate both earlier statute law and later case law in one statute.

To become an Act of Parliament, legislation must receive the approval of both Houses of Parliament (Lords and Commons) and it must also receive Royal Assent. A statute is presented to the House of Commons as a Bill. These take two forms. The first category involves Bills sponsored by the Government, which almost certainly will result in legislation if the Government has a majority. MPs are generally constrained to vote along party political lines. In addition, Government sponsored legislation is allocated a greater amount of parliamentary time. Alternatively, there may be Bills on which the Government allows its supporters a free vote so that they can make their decision on a point of conscience. An example is the Abortion Act 1967. The second main category are Private Members' Bills. These, as the name suggests, are Bills introduced into Parliament which do not have the sponsorship of the Government. These Bills will usually only become law if they have Government support.

A statute may provide an outline of the legal position but then leave provisions to be defined by later secondary legislation known as 'statutory instruments'. This enables the legislation to have a more rapid passage through Parliament. So for example, the Human Organ Transplants Act 1989 set down a regime for undertaking transplants from living organ donors, but the detailed procedure for undertaking those transplants was laid down in subsequent statutory instruments.

Government departments such as the Department of Health issue circulars. While such documents do not have the force of law, they may provide guidance as to what conduct constitutes accepted practice.

Statutory interpretation

A statute may state general legal obligations but where disputes later arise the statute will require interpretation. A court will examine the statute to see how it applies in a particular situation. A word or phrase within the statute may be ambiguous and require construction by the court. There are a number of rules of statutory interpretation that the court may apply. The court may look at the words of the statute and apply them literally. However, it is more likely that the court will construe a word or phrase in the light of the 'purpose' of the statute (Smith and Bailey 1996).

Common law

In some situations, there is no legislation governing a particular area, or if there is room for interpretation of the statute then it may be necessary to look elsewhere for guidance as to what is the current law. The relevant law may be found in common law, the term given to describe law which has arisen from previous decisions of the courts on that issue.

Precedent: Some cases are more important than others. Case law operates through a system of precedent. A later court may be obliged to follow the decision of an earlier court. The decisions of the highest court of the land, the House of Lords, are binding on all lower courts. Decisions of the Court of Appeal are also very important and generally bind lower courts. Where a case arises involving a very important point of law it may be referred up to the House of Lords in order to obtain a definitive ruling as to the legal position in this area. For example, the famous case of *Gillick* v. *West Norfolk and Wisbech AHA* which concerned the legality of providing children under 16 years of age with contraceptive advice and treatment without parental consent was heard in the High Court, the Court of Appeal and then in the House of Lords ([1985] 2 All ER 545).

The decisions of some lower courts do not act as binding precedents, for example, decisions at magistrates' court level. As far as tribunals are concerned, in theory each case is decided on its own facts. But tribunal decisions are frequently reported and as a consequence general principles have become established.

Interpreting cases: While there may not be a previous case with precisely the same facts, that does not mean that there are no previous cases which can be followed. Lawyers, when trying to discover the current law from previously decided cases, are primarily concerned not with the facts of a particular case, but with the point of law which was decided in that case - the *ratio decendendi*. They then use that point of law in order to argue by analogy to the particular case before them. In a particular case a judge may make a suggestion as to his or her view of the law, a statement which is not directly related to the decision in that case. That statement, known as the *obiter dictum* does not bind lower courts. However, an *obiter* statement may be referred to in a later case as providing a helpful judicial view on the point of law in question.

European law

In 1973 the United Kingdom signed the Treaty of Rome and entered the European Economic Community (EEC). Since then UK law has been increasingly affected by European law. In 1993 the Treaty of European Union was passed which created a new body - the European Union. This is comprised of the states of the European Community but is broader in scope than the EEC.

The European Community Act 1972 provides that rights created by or arising out of the Community Treaties shall have effect in UK law (s2(1) European Communities Act 1972). In addition we are affected by European secondary legislation; this is made up of regulations, directives and decisions. Regulations are binding and they are directly applicable in English law, which means that the English courts are required to apply such regulations in English cases. Directives are binding but generally each state is left to determine the manner in which they apply. However, directives do apply to state authorities without further incorporation and this includes NHS bodies (*Marshall* v. *Southampton and SW Hampshire AHA* [1986] ECR 723). There are many directives in the area of health and safety which have had a considerable impact upon nursing practice, such as the Control of Substances Hazardous to Health regulations (1988).

The European Court of Justice sits in Luxembourg. If in an English case point of law arises and a UK statute appears to be in conflict with European law, European law is supreme (*Van Gend en Loos* v. *Netherlands Belastingens-administratie* [1963] CMLR 105 ECJ). If there is uncertainty as to the extent to which, for example, a European directive applies in English law then a reference can be made to the European Court of Justice under a procedure known as Article 177, asking for their opinion on this case. Decisions made by the European Court of Justice may be directly binding on English courts and at the very least English courts will take notice of them (s2(1) European Communities Act 1972).

European Convention on Human Rights

We are also party to the European Convention of Human Rights. This is totally separate to our membership of the European Union. The

European Convention of Human Rights came into force on 3 September 1953. Individual citizens of the UK have had a right to petition under the Convention since 1966. The Convention contains a list of what are regarded as fundamental human rights. If a person believes that one of his or her fundamental rights has been violated and the claim is not upheld in the English courts, s/he can seek to bring the case before the European Commission of Human Rights in Strasbourg. It will investigate the claim and may refer the case to the European Court of Human Rights. Actions have been brought, for example challenging a woman's decision to have an abortion (*Paton* v. *UK* [1980] 3 EHRR 408). Where a claim is upheld before the European Court of Human Rights the English courts are not bound to follow it, nor is Parliament bound to change the law on that matter. But in practice, in most situations, the legislature responds to a finding at the European Court of Human Rights and may make a legislative change.

The nurse in the courtroom

When is the nurse likely to appear in court? S/he may be a party to an action so, for example, the nurse may be a plaintiff in a civil claim bringing an action for damages against her or his employer on the grounds of the employer's negligence. In a claim brought by a patient, the nurse may be called to give evidence; this may be as to what the nurse saw happen to a patient claiming that s/he was given negligent treatment. In addition, the nurse may be called to give expert evidence, for example in a negligence action as to the standard of practice which would be expected of a responsible nursing professional in that situation (see below).

Structure of health care provision

Most health care provided in England is provided by the NHS though nurses may of course work outside the NHS eg nursing homes and residential care homes (these are required to be registered under the Registered Homes Act 1984). In this section, the structure of health care provision within the NHS is examined. The Secretary of State for Health is accountable to Parliament for the operation of the health service. S/he controls NHS expenditure through the use of cash limits. Day to day management of the Health Service is undertaken by the NHS Executive (NHSE), which is largely based in Leeds.

The structure of the NHS has been altered by the Health Authorities Act 1995. Prior to 1 April 1996, below the NHSE in England were regional health authorities (RHAs). After that date RHAs were abolished, with their statutory functions being transferred to eight 'regional outposts' of the NHSE (Health Authorities Act 1995). These bodies are responsible for overseeing the efficient operation of the internal market.

Prior to 1 April 1996, below the regions health care was regulated through district health authorities (DHAs) and Family Health Service authorities (FHSAs). The Health Authorities Act 1995 introduced amendments to this structure. As of 1 April 1996 DHAs and FHSAs were merged to form new unitary health authorities. This is part of a movement towards greater focus on primary health care provision. General practitioners are under an obligation to provide care to those patients who are on their list. In addition, they are required to provide care to other persons seeking treatment where treatment is 'immediately required' (Terms and Conditions of Service, paragraph 4(1)b.)

Many nurses are employed by trusts or by general practitioners. Trusts, whether hospital or community, are run by boards of directors. They have a duty to undertake their functions efficiently, effectively and economically. A large number of community health services are now also trusts. In 1994, the Secretary of State for Health introduced a Code of Conduct and Accountability (NHSE EL (94) (40)). This Code requires that those who serve on NHS boards should declare any interests they have in NHS contracts and that an audit/remuneration committee is set up to examine payments made to board members.

In 1990, the National Health Service and Community Care Act created an 'internal market' in health care. Health care provision was to be purchased from 'providers'. Purchasers were to be DHA's and general practice fundholders (GPFH), and providers were to include the new National Health Service trusts (NHSTs) and also private hospitals. Parties within this internal market in health care enter into contracts. Contracts between NHS purchasers and private sector providers take a conventional legal form and are enforceable in the courts in the usual way. This meant little change from the position prior to 1990, as for many years DHAs had been buying some services from independent hospitals. However, after 1990, dealings between bodies within the NHS itself were to be operated via contracts. Contracts are placed between NHS bodies which have no direct management relationship. These cover arrangements such as those between a GPFH and a hospital and an NHST. The Act calls these 'NHS contracts'. Confusingly, despite their name, these contracts are not enforceable in the courts. Instead a special procedure has been established to which these disputes can be referred (s4(3)). There may be nursing input into contract negotiations and nursing representation on the contract negotiations team, although the extent of nursing involvement in purchasing decisions is variable.

Much emphasis is being placed upon standards in health care through documents such as the Patient's Charter. This document is essentially a list of guidelines. Breach of Patient Charter requirements are not directly enforceable in the courts, although the contents of the Patient's Charter may be influential as indicating standards of care. It is usual for contracts between health authorities and NHS trusts to require Patient Charter targets to be met. Provision of health care is also being monitored through medical audit and nursing audit.

Challenges to failure to provide health services

The Secretary of State for Health has various statutory duties. Section 1 of the National Health Service Act 1977 states:

> 'It is the Secretary of State's duty to continue the promotion in England and Wales of a comprehensive health service designed to ensure improvement :
> (a) in the physical and mental health of the people of those countries and
> (b) in the prevention, diagnosis and treatment of illness and for that purpose to provide or secure effective provision of services in accordance with the Act.'

Section 3 of that Act states:

> 'It is the Secretary of State's duty to provide throughout England and Wales to such extent as he considers necessary to meet all reasonable requirements - (a) hospital accommodation... (c) medical, dental, nursing and ambulance services... (f) such other services as are required for the diagnosis and treatment of illness.'

Can the Secretary of State be held liable if services are not provided? In a number of cases persons have challenged a failure to provide health care services in the courts. For example, patients in Birmingham challenged the health authority's refusal to provide a unit for orthopaedic services (*R* v. *Secretary of State for Social Service ex parte Hincks* (1980) (1979) 123 *Sol J* 436). The application failed. In the Court of Appeal, Lord Denning, agreeing with the judge at first instance, stated that the Secretary of State's duty needed to be read in the light of the financial resources which he had available. Subsequently, in two cases, both concerning surgery required on an infant, the courts again rejected the claim that in refusing to provide these facilities the Secretary of State had acted in breach of duty.

In the second case Stephen Brown L.J. stated that:

> 'this is a hearing before a court. This is not the forum in which a court can properly express opinions upon the way in which national resources are allocated or distributed. [There] may be very good reasons why the resources in this case do not allow all the beds in the hospital to be used at this particular time. We have no evidence of that and indeed... it is not for this court or for any other court to substitute its own judgment for the judgement of those who are responsible for the allocation of resources.'

It might have been thought that the advent of the NHS internal market would have led to more parties 'chancing their arm' on resource issues. However, litigants have not been flocking to the courts.

The question of allocation of resources arose in the context of a well publicised case involving a young child. B, a 10-year-old child, suffered from leukaemia. Treatment was undertaken involving chemotherapy and a bone marrow transplant which was initially successful; however, the cancer recurred. Cambridgeshire Health Authority refused to authorise a further course of treatment. Doctors stated that a third course of chemotherapy and a further transplant would not be in the child's best interests and that, overall, the success rate of the procedure was 1-4%. The child's father sought to challenge the decision to refuse treatment. The case was heard first in the High Court and then on appeal in the Court of Appeal (*R* v. *Cambridge District Health Authority ex parte B* [1995] 2 All ER 129). Both hearings took place on the same afternoon.

At first instance in the High Court, Laws J. said that in determining whether to give treatment, the Health Authority must act reasonably. This meant that in making the decision, the Health Authority should have regard to all relevant considerations. In this case he said the Health Authority had not taken into consideration the views of B's family. He was also of the view that in a situation where, as here, a patient was at risk of death, the Health Authority had to explain why it had decided not to fund the treatment.

However, his judgment was overturned in the Court of Appeal. Sir Thomas Bingham, the Master of the Rolls held that, while the Finance Director of the Health Authority had not spoken directly to the family he had noted the interests of the family. In addition, difficult issues concerning resource allocation had to be weighed in the balance. He stated that:

> 'Difficult and agonising judgements had to be made as to how a limited budget could best be allocated for the maximum advantage of the maximum number of patients. That was not a judgment for the court.'

Sir Thomas Bingham held that the Authority had weighed up the various factors in reaching the decision and had not acted unreasonably. Relevant factors were that the treatment was untested and that it could almost be regarded as being experimental in its nature. There was only around a 1-4% success rate. In addition, the court noted the fact that there were potentially dehabilitating side effects. The court held that in these circumstances the decision of the health authority was not unreasonable.

Thus the courts are still unlikely to scrutinise resource allocation questions. Even if they were prepared to intervene, it is arguable that the courts do not provide an appropriate forum for such scrutiny. The whole question of rationing in health care needs to be addressed at national level rather than on a case by case basis as matters are referred to the courts. We may profit from consideration of the model adopted in one USA state, Oregon, where rationing has been put on a statutory footing (Newdick,

1995). Here, public consultation was undertaken before a list of treatment priorities was enacted in statute.

Professional accountability

The work of nurses in this country is overseen by their professional governing body, the UKCC, which is established by the Nurses, Midwives and Health Visitors Act 1997. The UKCC is composed of a council containing a maximum of sixty members (s1 Nurses, Midwives and Health Visitors Act 1997). Two thirds are registered nurses, midwives or health visitors elected from their professional peers. One third are appointed by Government ministers after consultation with bodies including professional organisations and consumer groups. They are health professionals or persons with experience in other fields, such as education, which are believed by the Secretary of State to be appropriate.

The UKCC keeps a register of nurses, midwives and health visitors (s7 Nurses, Midwives and Health Visitors Act 1997). There are 15 subcategories to the register, e.g. children's nurses and mental illness. It establishes rules regarding entry, removal and reinstatement from the register. Qualifications obtained in other European community countries will be recognised and the UKCC also recognises other qualifications. Nurses may be entered on the register if they have an appropriate professional qualification and are of good character. The UKCC is also concerned with nurse training, both at entry into the profession and post-qualification (S2 1997 Act). The UKCC provides guidance as to what are acceptable standards of professional conduct through its Code of Conduct and other statements such as its Guidelines for Professional Practice (UKCC, 1996a). As the reader will see later, the nurse may face a difficult dilemma if her or his obligations under the professional ethical code and under the contract of employment are at variance.

If a nurse is found to have behaved in a manner which constitutes 'misconduct' then s/he is liable to disciplinary action (s10 Nurses, Midwives and Health Visitors Act 1997). The Rules define misconduct as being 'conduct unworthy of a nurse, midwife or health visitor (Rule 1(2)).' Initial allegations are screened by an officer of the UKCC. There may be a short investigation by a solicitor to establish whether there is a case to answer. The matter may then be referred to the Preliminary Proceedings Committee. The Committee examines allegations made against practitioners. If it finds that these are trivial it may 'decline to proceed'. If, however, it takes the view that the allegations concern a matter which is probably misconduct, then this can be referred for a formal public hearing. Alternatively, the Committee may direct the Registrar to issue a formal caution (s11 Nurses, Midwives and Health Visitors Act 1997 and rule 4 SI 1993) if the charges are admitted. The Committee may also convene a hearing as a matter of urgency and order that a practitioner be suspended prior to a formal hearing before the Professional Conduct Committee (rule 3 of Professional Conduct Rules).

Serious matters are referred to the Professional Conduct Committee. This Committee considers cases and makes findings on the basis that professional misconduct has been proven beyond all reasonable doubt. The practitioner may choose to be represented by a lawyer/trade union officer, etc (Rule 13(5)). Where allegations are not admitted a hearing with cross-examination of witnesses is undertaken. The Committee has a number of powers. A name can be removed from the register, the practitioner may be issued with a caution (rules 9 and 18), the Committee may postpone judgement for a fixed period (rule 18), or a decision may be made to take no action. It should be noted that after a finding of misconduct has been made but before sanction is determined the committee should hear evidence as to the nurse's general record and the nurse may cross-examine witnesses and challenge any new allegations (Rule 18(3)). Grounds for removal include abuse of patients, breach of confidentiality and 'reckless and wilfully unskilled practice' (UKCC 1990) also failure to provide training to a nurse who requested it and breach of other managerial responsibilities.

The nurse has the right to appeal from either of these committees to the High Court (s12 Nurses, Midwives and Health Visitors Act 1997). However, in practice the court is unlikely to overturn the decision, as they are more prepared to accept the professional judgment (*Slater* v. *UKCC* unreported 18 May 1988 (QBD)). In addition, the conduct of proceedings of the committee may be subject to judicial review. The committees are under a duty to act fairly and must give nurses an opportunity to present their case and to answer the charges made against them. If they fail to do so, this may lead to a challenge that the conduct of the hearing was contrary to the rules of natural justice (*Hefferen* v. *The Committee of the UKCC* (1988); *The Independent*, 11 March).

A nurse who has been removed from the register may later apply to be restored (Rule 22). A hearing is held at which the nurse is entitled to be present. The nurse must nominate two persons to act as referees. These must be persons with knowledge of the facts and who have known the nurse since s/he was removed from the register. The UKCC has recently indicated that it is tightening up the grounds on which individuals may be restored to the register. This followed controversy over the restoration of two persons who had originally been removed when they had been convicted for rape. Applications to restore to the register will be heard every 4 months. These will be heard by a panel of four, usually chaired by the president of the UKCC and one panel member will be drawn from a consumer organisation. The UKCC has stated that 'for certain offences such as murder, rape, child abuse and serious physical assault, the applicant will not be restored to the register if this is likely to undermine public confidence in the professions regulated by the UKCC' (UKCC, 1996b).

Illness: If a Committee examining a claim of professional misconduct believes that the matter raised concerns a question of ill health then it may be referred to a separate panel, the Health Committee (Rule 29). Initially, such a claim is considered by professional screeners (Rule 9(3)). They may refer the claim to the Health Committee or, alternatively, decide that it concerns matters outside the remit of that Committee and that it should be referred back to the Professional Conduct Committee. The Health Committee examines whether the nurse's ability to practise has been seriously impaired by a physical or mental condition. If the Committee believes that her or his ability is so impaired then it must ban the nurse from practising. The Committee must order that the nurse be removed or suspended from the register (Rules 3,5).

Midwives: Midwives are also subject to further regulation through local supervisors who are appointed by the local supervising authority (s15 Nurses, Midwives and Health Visitors Act 1997). Midwives are required to inform supervisors of where they intend to practise. Supervisors can investigate or suspend midwives if they present a risk to public health because they could spread illness or because of misconduct (Rule 38).

The National Boards: In addition the UKCC bodies known as National Boards appointed by the Secretary of State have a role regulating nursing. There are three Boards (one each for England, Wales and Scotland). The Boards comprise a chief executive and six appointed members including one representative from each of the professions (s5 1997 Act). In the past they were involved in regulating misconduct but today their role is more limited. They have the task of approving institutions providing training courses for nurses, midwives and health visitors (s6 1997 Act).

Conclusions

This chapter has set out the framework of regulation within which the nurse undertakes her or his practice. In subsequent chapters the operation of the law is considered in a number of areas which are particularly pertinent to nursing practice.

References

Bailey, S.H. and Gunn, M.J. (1996) *Smith and Bailey on the English Legal System.* Sweet and Maxwell, London (Chapter 6).

Newdick, C. (1995) *Who Should We Treat?* Oxford University Press, Oxford, pp. 30-36.

Nurses, Midwives and Health Visitors (Professional Conduct Rules) 1993 SI 1993 No. 893.

Tingle, J. and Cribb, A. (eds) (1995) *Nursing Law and Ethics.* Blackwell Scientific Publications, Oxford.

UKCC (1996a) *Guidelines for Professional Practice.* UKCC, London.

UKCC (1996b) UKCC tightens its rules on restorations to the register. *Register*, **17**, 3.

UKCC (1992) *Scope of Professional Practice.* United Kingdom Central Council for Nursing, Midwifery and Health Visiting, London.

UKCC (1990) 'With a view to removal from the register'. UKCC, London.

Woolf, Lord. (1996) *Access to Justice.* HMSO, London.

Chapter 2

Nursing negligence: General issues

John Tingle

Introduction

Nurses are not only professionally accountable to patients through the United Kingdom Central Council for Nursing, Midwifery and Health Visiting (UKCC) Code of Professional Conduct, but like all other professionals they are accountable in law and malpractice may lead to a civil action or a criminal prosecution. A nurse is under a legal duty to act carefully towards the patient. If a nurse fails to exercise sufficient care and by so doing causes injury or harm to the patient, s/he will be held liable in the tort of negligence.

The next section considers liability in tort for negligent conduct; later sections consider liability in criminal law where actions are gravely negligent, and some issues regarding reform of the law of negligence. The present chapter focuses upon general principles of liability. Various related negligence issues are examined in later chapters, including liability under certain statutes for negligence. Liability where injury arises from defective drugs is discussed in the context of nurse prescribing in Chapter 4. Issues of liability of injury caused by defective products to both nurses and patients are considered in Chapter 9, while questions of liability in relation to childbirth and conception are considered in Chapter 11.

Liability in tort for negligent conduct

Accidents sometimes happen

A nurse is not negligent if s/he acts in accordance with a practice accepted as proper by a responsible body of nursing opinion. The nurse is not expected to take precautions against unforeseeable risks and even if risks are foreseeable they may still be justified in the particular circumstances of the case. Accidents, untoward incidents or adverse treatment outcomes may occur without any findings of fault being made against the nurse. The following two examples illustrate this point.

A competent nurse, following the correct procedure for venipuncture, may still cause the patient to develop a haematoma, or bleed after the removal of the needle if the patient is on anticoagulant therapy. This may happen occasionally even though the nurse has ascertained that the patient is taking anticoagulants and applied pressure to the site of venipuncture her- or himself. Bruising can be reduced if pressure is applied by the nurse or phlebotomist, but bruising can still occur in the older patient and, occasionally, slight pain and discomfort.

Ribs have been known to fracture when a patient receives external cardiac massage when the nurse has carried out the procedure correctly.

Elements of the tort of negligence

Generally speaking, the plaintiff (the person bringing the court action) must prove negligence against the nurse or the nurse's employers. The plaintiff will normally have to prove his case on the 'balance of probabilities' (Montgomery, 1995). The elements of the tort of negligence must be established. The basic elements are as follows:

- Duty
- Breach
- Damage
- Remoteness.

Duty

The plaintiff must firstly establish that the defendant (nurse or health authority, trust) owed him a legal duty of care. In the health care context this is usually not a problem as Jones (1992) has commented when defining the tort:

> 'In cases of medical negligence the existence of a duty owed to the patient is usually regarded as axiomatic, and attention normally focuses on whether there has been a breach of duty or whether the breach caused damage.'

However, the issue of duty could problematic where a nurse acts as a 'Good Samaritan' and causes further injury by negligently administering first aid to the accident victim.

The courts are unlikely to find an express legal duty to rescue a stranger; the nurse could walk past the victim with legal impunity (Tingle, 1991). However, if the nurse stops and acts then a legal duty of care will flow from her or his actions. The nurse now could be sued if s/he practices first aid negligently and causes further injury. In contrast, it appears that in some instances the UKCC would expect the nurse to act as a Good Samaritan and assist if s/he could easily do so. Examples 2 and 3 given by the UKCC in their recent advisory document (UKCC, 1996) provide useful illustrations of the UKCC approach to the nurse as Good Samaritan. In example 3 (see Appendix 1 section 14) a distinction is made between legal and professional duties. A nurse would be expected to make some response in the emergency situation postulated, at the very least comforting and supporting the injured patient. There is a risk, however, that if s/he does act and make a mistake then legal consequences may follow. However, it should be remembered that the likelihood of a Good Samaritan being sued is fairly remote and that the public interest is better served by doing and encouraging Good Samaritan acts.

Duty questions

The first issue is whether a person has in fact become a patient of a health care professional or a hospital. This question is discussed in sections 11-14 of UKCC (UKCC 1996) and some useful illustrations are given. The following situation may also help to explain the issue:

An injured confused man wanders into a hospital after a road traffic accident and is unable to locate the accident and emergency department. He requires urgent medical treatment. A hospital security guard passes him in a corridor in the hospital and does not challenge or question him. A nurse hurrying home after finishing her shift also passes him without stopping. Should the guard and the nurse have stopped and questioned him?

Can the guard and the nurse be said to have owed a duty of care to the accident victim which would have required such action? Furthermore, what about the position of the hospital? Were there any organisational failures, such as failure to erect a signpost properly or to man a reception desk, which would make the hospital directly liable for any negligence?

Much will depend on the circumstances of the case and on answers to factual questions such as: how ill did the victim look?; what was the time of the incident?; and so on. It will be seen that Example 2 of section 14 UKCC (1996) is similar in facts to the problem discussed. The UKCC states that in its example the nurse would be expected to take some action, comforting and supporting the patient and calling for expert help.

Breach

The second step is for the plaintiff to prove that the nurse was negligent; in breach of her or his legal duty of care. The nurse's conduct would be viewed from the perspective of what 'the ordinary skilled nurse in her speciality would have done in the circumstances of the case'. The nurse would also have been expected to take precautions against reasonably known risks only.

Legal standard of nursing competence

In determining the legal standard of care if litigation was being brought, lawyers would have to take advice from other nurses in the same speciality.

If the case went to trial, the judge would hear expert evidence and would draw conclusions from this as to the standard of professional practice. The legal principles stated come from the well known *Bolam* case (*Bolam* v. *Friern Hospital Management Committee* [1957] 1 WLR 582). In the case, the Judge, Mr Justice McNair, stated what has become known as the *Bolam* test:

> 'The test is the standard of the ordinary skilled man exercising and professing to have that special skill. A man need not possess the highest expert skill; it is well established law that it is sufficient if he exercises the ordinary skill of an ordinary competent man exercising that particular art...'

The judge went on to say that a professional would not be liable in negligence:

> '...if he has acted in accordance with a practice accepted as proper by a responsible body of medical men skilled in that particular art...Putting it the other way round, a man is not negligent, if he is acting in accordance with such a practice, merely because there is a body of opinion who would take a contrary view.'

Sections 15 and 16 of UKCC (1996) provide a discussion of the concept of reasonableness with reference to the *Bolam* principle (see Legal standard of nursing competence section above). If a nurse is a trainee s/he is still expected to accord with the standard of a qualified practitioner (*Nettleship* v. *Weston* [1971] 2 QB 691). Nurses who are unsure of what to do should get advice from a more experienced practitioner. By doing so, not only are they acting in accordance with good practice but this is likely to absolve them of liability in negligence (*Wilsher* v. *Essex AHA* [1986]3 All ER 801).

Reasonable differences of opinion

There may be legitimate differences as to what constitutes a body of responsible professional practice. Take, for instance, the issue of nurses using cot-sides. One nurse may decide to use cot-sides while another nurse may refuse to have them on her or his ward because it is known patients can roll over the sides and fall from a higher level. Another nurse may decide not to take any of these courses of action and decide to nurse the patient on a mattress on the floor. Nursing experts advising lawyers and the court would say that, generally speaking, all the above nursing actions are reasonable and that there are competent bodies of nursing opinion which would support such practices. Applying the *Bolam* test the courts would usually accept the nursing experts' views and would not choose between competing views and practices. A small number of medical practitioners could constitute a responsible body of medical opinion (*De Freitas* v. *O'Brien and Another*.([1993] 4 Med LR 281).

The courts have not handed over totally the job of determining the standard of care to the nursing and medical professions. While expert evidence as to nursing or medical practice will usually be accepted, the courts could still overrule a body of professional practice. Nevertheless, the courts would not easily condemn accepted nursing or medical practice as negligent (Jones, 1996). The question of what happens when professional opinion differs was considered by the House of Lords in a case involving a nurse plaintiff (*Maynard* v. *West Midlands Regional Health Authority* ([1984] 1 WLR 634)). Staff Nurse Maynard consulted a physician and a surgeon experienced in the treatment of chest diseases. Tuberculosis was considered to be the most likely diagnosis, but there were symptoms which also suggested Hodgkin's disease, carcinoma and sarcoidosis. Unless there was early treatment of Hodgkin's disease it would prove fatal (as treatment was understood in 1970). The doctors decided upon a mediastinoscopy, which would provide them with a biopsy which they could have examined immediately. The operation involved a risk of damage to the left laryngeal nerve even if carried out correctly. Unfortunately, the nerve was damaged despite the fact that the operation was carried out carefully. The biopsy proved negative and it was later confirmed that the plaintiff was suffering from tuberculosis and not Hodgkin's disease. She sued in negligence alleging, amongst other things, that it was a negligent decision to carry out the mediastinoscopy rather than await the results of the sputum test. Her action failed. Lord Scarman stated:

> 'A case which is based on an allegation that a fully considered decision of two consultants in the field of their special skill was negligent clearly presents certain difficulties of proof. It is not enough to show that there is a body of competent professional opinion which considers that theirs was a wrong decision, if there also exists a body of professional opinion, equally competent, which supports the decision as reasonable in the circumstances. It is not enough to show that subsequent events show that the operation need never have been performed, if at the time the decision to operate was taken it was reasonable in the sense that a responsible body of medical opinion would have accepted it as proper...Differences of opinion and practice exist, and will always exist, in the medical as in other professions. There is seldom any one answer exclusive of all others to problems of professional judgement.'

These legal principles can be applied to another controversial nursing issue; the Edinburgh University solution of lime (Eusol) wound care dressing debate (Tingle, 1990). Many nurses are reluctant to use Eusol, with some arguing that they have a professional duty not to do so as they say it is ineffective as a promoter of wound healing. Some consultants like to use Eusol and ask nurses to use it. There have been a number of publicised disputes as nurses face a conflict between the consultants request and their own professional view on Eusol. Applying the principles set out in *Bolam* and *Maynard* it can be seen that, generally speaking, it is not negligent to use Eusol because there is a competent body of medical opinion which would support its use (Burton, 1993).

Developments in health care practice generally may influence the manner in which the *Bolam* test may operate, and assist in defining what amounts to a responsible body of professional practice. It is interesting to speculate the extent to which concepts such as evidenced based medicine/nursing and clinical guidelines and protocols will push the standard of care, from reasonable practice in the *Bolam* sense, to best practice. Evidence based medicine is practice based on a clear body of research and agreed principles. The *Bolam* test may also be affected by standards of practice such as requirements of information disclosure, which may be imposed by parties entering into NHS contracts (Barker, 1995). It is also unclear whether nurses will be subject to the same degree of scrutiny as doctors, or indeed whether the courts would be willing to undertake a more rigorous review than is the case as regards medical decision making.

Departing from accepted practice

A nurse would not necessarily be viewed as being negligent if s/he departed from accepted nursing practice in a particular situation. For example, a wound care specialist might decide, on the basis of a recent research study, to mix two types of topical wound care solutions together and apply them to a patient's wound, arguing that recent research has shown that when the solutions are mixed together they became more effective. This is not, however, the conventional way to apply the solutions. If problems do occur and the patient then takes legal action, the nurse would have to justify the departure from conventional practice. There is a clear danger in accepting claims made by *one* research paper only. There is a need for confirmation and exploration of the implications of changing practice. There must be critical appraisal of new research.

If a nurse is given instructions by a doctor but is of the view that these are wrong, what should s/he do? It is suggested that it would be good practice to raise the concerns with the doctor. But if the doctor disagrees and the nurse goes along with the doctor's instructions, then if harm results the nurse is likely to be held not negligent because s/he was acting on doctor's orders (*Gold* v. *Essex County Council* [1942] 2 All ER 237; Montgomery, 1995).

Assessing risk

The nurse in the above example might have felt that there were no real significant adverse risks to the patient in her or his proposed course of action, the benefits outweighing any treatment risks. Whether the nurse was correct in her or his assessment would be an important issue for the experts to determine in their reports to the lawyers.

Taking precautions against foreseeable risks

The defendant's conduct in a negligence case is viewed from the date the incident occurred and not from the time of the court hearing. The defendant would be expected only to guard against events which could be reasonably foreseen at the time of the alleged negligence. *Roe* v. *Ministry of Health and Others*, *Woolley* v. *Same* ([1954] 2 ALL ER 131) illustrates this point. Two patients underwent an operation. Prior to the operation a spinal anaesthetic consisting of Nupercaine was administered to the patients by a lumbar puncture. The plaintiffs developed spastic paraplegia after the operation and were paralysed from the waist down. Their injuries were caused by the injection of contaminated Nupercaine. The Nupercaine was in glass ampoules which, prior to administration, were immersed in a phenol solution. Unknown to the anaesthetist, the phenol had percolated into the glass ampoules by means of invisible cracks or molecular flaws in the glass. At the time of the incident, the risk of percolation in the manner that occurred was not generally appreciated by competent anaesthetists. It was an unforeseeable occurrence. The defendants were not legally expected to anticipate the danger. Denning L.J. expressed the following sentiment in the case, which can equally be said to be applicable to all health care professionals today:

> 'Every surgical operation is attended by risks. We cannot take the benefits without taking the risks. Every advance in technique is also attended by risks. Doctors, like the rest of us, have to learn by experience; and experience often teaches in a hard way. Something goes wrong and shows up a weakness, and then it is put right. That is just what happened here...we must not look at the 1947 accident with 1954 spectacles.'

Legal duty to keep up to date

A nurse could breach her or his legal duty of care by not keeping up to date with major developments in her or his speciality. Consider the following example. A new wound care dressing has been created which is very effective and is becoming widely used. A district nurse is unaware of the new dressing because she feels she has no time to read the professional journals or attend study days which are put on by her employer at regular intervals. One of her patients has a wound which will not heal. Another district nurse attends the patient and uses the new dressing and the wound heals very quickly. The patient asks why the new dressing was not used before by the regular district nurse.

This issue is addressed by the UKCC in the *Code of Professional Conduct* (1992i):

> 'As a registered nurse, midwife or health visitor, you are personally accountable for your practice and, in the exercise of your professional accountability, must...maintain and improve your professional knowledge and competence.'

The nurse in the wound care example, as well as possibly being in breach of her duty of care to her patient, could also be viewed as being in breach of clause 3 of the *Code of Professional Conduct* (UKCC, 1992i): blind indifference to her professional duty of personal updating and development. She should try to keep reasonably up to date.

Within the nursing profession the Clinical Supervision initiative and the UKCC Post-Registration Education and Practice Project (PREP) provides an important professional impetus for personal updating. The issue of professional updating has been considered by the Court of Appeal in *Crawford* v. *Board of Governors of Charing Cross Hospital* (1953) (*The Times*, 8 December 1953). The plaintiff Mr Robert Joseph Crawford was admitted to the Charing Cross Hospital for an operation for the removal of his bladder. The plaintiff's left arm was extended at an angle from his body so that a blood transfusion could be given. After the operation the plaintiff complained of paralysis in his left arm; brachial palsy had developed. He sued alleging negligence. The main issue was whether the anaesthetist was negligent in missing an article which appeared in *The Lancet* in January 1950; the operation was performed in July 1950. The article warned about the risk of brachial palsy when the arm was kept in an extended position. The plaintiff did not succeed as no negligence was found. Denning LJ states that all reasonable care was taken by the hospital and that it would amount to imposing too high a burden on the doctor to require that he read all articles in the medical press.

The judgement on the facts makes sense; nobody can read all the professional articles which appear in the numerous journals. Nonetheless, while ignorance of one warning in the professional press may be acceptable, missing a number of warnings could well lead to a finding of negligence. Mason and McCall Smith (1994i), referring to the *Crawford* case, feel that a less charitable view would be taken if the same facts occurred today:

> 'The practice of medicine has, however, become increasingly based on principles of scientific elucidation and report and the pressure on doctors to keep abreast of current developments is now considerable. It is no longer possible for a doctor to coast along on the basis of long experience; as in many professions and callings, such an attitude has been firmly discredited.'

The courts have recently affirmed the health care professional's obligation to keep her- or himself up to date by familiarity with mainstream literature (*Gascoine* v. *Ian Shendan and Co and Lathan* [1994] 5 Med LR 437).

The nurse must thus remember the professional and legal duty to keep up to date with developments in nursing practice.

Damage

The plaintiff must prove that the defendant's breach of duty caused or materially contributed to his or her damage. A direct link has to be made between the two elements of breach and damage. The plaintiff must b 'able to prove that the negligence has made a difference, that it has adversely affected the condition in some way'. A first step is to prove factual causation: the cause *in fact* of the plaintiff's condition.

Causation in fact

Lawyers use a test known as the 'but for test'. Jones (1991i) summarises this test as follows:

> 'The first step is to eliminate irrelevant causes, and this is the purpose of the 'but for test'. If harm to the plaintiff would not have occurred 'but for' the defendant's negligence then that negligence is a cause of the harm. It is not necessarily the cause because there may well be other events which are causally relevant. Putting this another way, if the loss would have been incurred in any event, the defendant's conduct is not a cause.'

The application of this principle can be illustrated by the case of *Barnett* v. *Chelsea and Kensington Hospital Management Committee* ([1968] 1 All ER 1068). The plaintiff, William Barnett, was a night-watchman at a college hall of residence. He was drinking some tea with two other night-watchmen. Soon afterwards they all started vomiting and went to the defendant's casualty department. They were seen by a nurse who telephoned the casualty officer, Dr Banerjee, who unfortunately was not feeling well himself. He did not see the men, saying that they should go home and see their own doctors. Mr Whittall, one of the men, was asked by Dr Banerjee to stay for an X-ray. He had seen Dr Banerjee on another matter sometime before. All the men went away and, some hours later, the plaintiff died. It was discovered later that the cause of death was arsenical poisoning. His widow claimed that the hospital had been negligent in not treating her husband. The casualty officer was found by the court to be in breach of his legal duty of care in not examining and treating Mr Barnett, but the legal action failed. Element 3, Causation in Fact, had not been proved; death had been inevitable for Mr Barnett. Had he been seen and admitted to hospital he would have died before the antidote could have been given. The defendant's breach of duty had, therefore, not caused his death; they could not have done anything to save him in time.

The plaintiff has the burden of proving that the defendant's actions or omissions have caused or materially contributed to the damage s/he has suffered. This can be a difficult task in medical and nursing negligence cases where there can often be a number of biological causes, natural causes of a plaintiff's condition. The burden of proof is on the plaintiff to establish that the breach of duty was a material contribution to the damage caused (*Wilsher* v. *Essex Area Health Authority* ([1986] 3 All ER 801). A nurse who is expert in the relevant speciality would be called to give evidence. A number of reported cases involve allegations of both medical and nursing negligence and in such circumstances both types of experts will be used.

The case of *Kay* v. *Ayrshire and Arran Health Board* [1987] 2 All ER 417 illustrates key causation principles. Andrew Stuart Kay was aged 2 years and 5 months when he was admitted to the Seafield Children's Hospital, Ayr. His GP admitted him because she thought he may have been suffering from meningitis and this diagnosis was later confirmed by the hospital. The consultant paediatrician in charge of the case instructed that 10 000 units of penicillin be administered intrathecally. By mistake, a senior house officer injected 300 000 units of penicillin instead of the required 10 000 units. Andrew went into convulsions and later developed a degree of paralysis on one side of his body. Immediate action was taken to remedy this negligent mistake. Andrew recovered and appeared to suffer no immediate ill-effects of the overdose. He made a rapid recovery from meningitis.

However, some time after his discharge from hospital his parents noticed that he appeared to be suffering from deafness; this was later confirmed. An action for negligence was commenced alleging that the overdose of penicillin had caused his deafness. The action failed because factual causation was not established: it could not be proven that the overdose caused or materially contributed to Andrew's deafness. The weight of evidence in the case pointed to the deafness being caused by the meningitis.

Bolitho: A case too far?

The case of *Bolitho* v. *City and Hackney Health Authority* (1993) 13 BMLR 111 has clouded the generally accepted principles of causation discussed above. The Court of Appeal, it has been argued, wrongly applied the *Bolam* test to the issue of factual causation (Kennedy and Grubb, 1993). In this case a 2-year-old boy was being treated for breathing difficulties in hospital. He suffered, on one day, two episodes of acute shortness of breath and a doctor was urgently summoned by the ward sister. The doctor failed to attend or arrange another doctor to attend. Later that day, the boy suffered a respiratory and cardiac arrest. He was resuscitated and was found to have brain damage. The health authority was sued for negligence. It was alleged that the plaintiff's brain damage was caused by the negligent failure of medical staff to attend.

Negligence was admitted by the defendants; medical staff should have attended when summoned, but that was not the end of the matter. Intubation of an infant is not an easy or completely safe procedure. The doctor who had been summoned and failed to attend said that she would not have intubated him even if she had attended. Expert opinion was divided on the necessity of intubation. The trial judge found for the health authority that causation had not been established applying the test outlined in the *Bolam* and *Maynard* cases. The doctor would not have intubated the plaintiff even if she had attended him; this was a course of action supported by a responsible body of medical opinion even though other doctors disagreed. The court would not choose between these competing though responsible views. The plaintiff appealed unsuccessfully to the Court of Appeal. This decision could be criticised on the ground that it further advances professional medical practice as the determinative factor in medical negligence actions.

Remoteness

Having established what factually caused the plaintiff's damage, there may still be a need to consider the cause for attributing legal responsibility, often termed remoteness, causation in law or proximate cause. A defendant generally cannot be held liable for everything that happens to a plaintiff; the damage may be too remote, outside the bounds of what can be legally recovered. Instances would be where the damage would be much more extensive, or of a different type, or occur in a different way, than would normally have been expected.

Example

A district nurse makes regular visits to an elderly patient to change dressings. The elderly patient lives alone and looks forward to the nurse's regular visits. The nurse gives her company and spends some of her time talking generally to the patient. Due to promotion the nurse needs to move districts, with another nurse taking over her visits. The patient appears to take this news well but the next day is found dead with a suicide note. The patient, unable to face the change in nursing routine, has committed suicide. The patient's relatives blame the nurse, saying that she should have anticipated the patient's reaction and taken preventative steps.

A key issue would be the foreseeability of the patient's action. Was there any existing evidence of psychiatric illness and was this passed on to the nurse? If there was no such evidence then it could be argued that the patient's actions would not have been reasonably foreseen by the nurse. She would not have been expected to act to prevent the suicide. The event would have been legally too remote.

In some situations there is more than one cause of harm which a patient suffers. Consider a patient who has been negligently knocked off his motorbike by a motorist. He is seriously injured with damage to the spine. The doctor in casualty causes further injury and paralysis through negligent medical treatment. In ascertaining legal liability, the court would have to consider evidence as to what caused the ultimate injury. It may be the case that both the motorist and doctor could be negligent and liable to some extent.

Where there are two or more defendants liable for the same damage to the plaintiff, the Civil Liability (Contribution) Act 1978 allows them to claim contributions from each other for any damages awarded.

Damages for loss of chance

What if there is a delay in providing treatment and the patient later seeks to bring an action, claiming that it was this delay which resulted in him or her not having a full recovery? In effect, the claim is that the negligence led to the 'loss of a chance' of recovery in that situation. This issue arose in the case of *Hotson* v. *East Berkshire Area Health Authority* ([1987] 2 All ER 909). The plaintiff was 13 years of age when he injured his hip in a fall. He had sustained an acute traumatic fracture of the left femoral epiphysis, but this condition was not diagnosed at the hospital when he attended and he was sent home. He was in severe pain for 5 days. He returned to the hospital and his condition was correctly diagnosed. He suffered avascular necrosis of the epiphysis. At the age of 20 years he had a major permanent disability.

The plaintiff claimed damages for negligence against the health authority, which admitted a breach of duty but denied that the resulting delay had adversely affected the plaintiff's long term condition. When the action was tried the trial judge found that even if the hospital medical staff had correctly diagnosed and treated the plaintiff on his first visit to the hospital there was still a 75% risk of the disability developing. The medical staff's breach of duty had turned that risk into an inevitability. The plaintiff was in effect denied a 25% chance of a good recovery. Damages were awarded which included an amount which represented 25% of the full value of the damages awardable for the disability. The Court of Appeal affirmed the judge's decision. The health authority successfully appealed to the House of Lords and the Court of Appeal's decision was reversed. The appeal was allowed on the narrow ground that the plaintiff failed to establish a cause of action in respect of the avascular necrosis and its consequences. The trial judge's finding of fact was that on the balance of probabilities the injury caused by the plaintiff's fall left insufficient blood vessels intact to keep the epiphysis alive. The fall was the sole cause of the avascular necrosis.

This case again graphically illustrates the practical difficulties in establishing causation. The broad issue raised by the case of the possibility of claiming for loss of chance in tort was left open by the House of Lords and it remains to be seen whether such an action may succeed in the future.

Res ipsa loquitur

There are circumstances when the courts are prepared to infer from the facts that a defendant was negligent. Under this evidential rule the burden of proof is not formally reversed and the inference of negligence can be rebutted. Generally speaking, the principle will apply where it is obvious that there has been negligence, for example, where the doctor has amputated the wrong leg or a swab or forceps has been left in a patient, etc. An extreme example of *res ipsa loquitur* was noted in the *Yorkshire Evening Post*, 14 October 1982:

> 'An enquiry has begun at a hospital in Vienna into how a man, suffering from a broken leg, was mistakenly given a heart pacemaker (Dixon, 1984).'

Further examples of situations in which *res ipsa loquitur* may be pleaded are to be found in the following cases cited by Action for Victims of Medical Accidents (AVMA):

> 'Foreign bodies were as varied as ever - ranging from swabs (14), insoluble sutures (5), clips (4), metal thread/wool (3), packs (3), bits of catheter apparatus (3), needles (2), clamps (2), gauze (2), scissors (1), forceps (1), and even part of a glass test tube. Most of these arose from abdominal surgery - 13 from gastroenterology cases. (AVMA, 1984-85i)'

The MDU (1993) noted a case where a patient received approximately £27 000 in compensation for an overlooked swab. This, in common with the other examples of the situation in which *res ipsa loquitur* might be used, can be seen to be of particular relevance to theatre nursing.

A number of conditions must be satisfied before the *res ipsa loquitur* principle can apply. The event, when it occurred, must have been under the control, supervision or management of the defendant. The event would not normally have happened unless there was negligence. The whole circumstances of the case would be considered. The lawyers and the judge would consider, as a matter of common sense and common experience, whether such events could have occurred without negligence. The defendant must have offered no reasonable explanation of what has happened.

The principle has worked in a number of health care cases. *Cassidy* v. *Ministry of Health* ([1951] 1 All ER 574) and *Bull* v. *Devon Area Health Authority* ([1989] [1993] 4 Med LR 117, 22 BMLR, 79) are just two cases where the principle has been used. In *Cassidy* the plaintiff was operated on for Dupuytren's contraction. He was suffering from a contraction of the third and fourth fingers of the left hand. After the operation, a nurse bandaged the plaintiff's hand and arm to a splint. The bandage was tested by a doctor to see if it was too tight; circulation was judged to be satisfactory. The patient subsequently complained of exceptional pain and was seen on occasions by medical staff. The splint and bandage were left intact and morphia was administered. The plaintiff continued to complain about excessive pain until the removal of the splint, when he discovered that he had lost the use of all four fingers. He sued for negligence in regard to the postoperational treatment he received. Even though he could not identify who in particular was negligent, the principle of *res ipsa loquitur* was applied. The evidence showed a *prima facie* case of negligence and this evidence was not rebutted by the defendants who were responsible for the medical and nursing staff.

Bull v. *Devon Area Health Authority* ([1989] [1993] 4 Med LR 117) demonstrates a controversial application of the principle; not all the judges in the case agreed to it being used. The case concerned the negligent organisation of maternity services. Mrs Bull was in premature labour carrying uniovular twins. The twins were sharing the same placenta. The first twin, later named Darryl, was spontaneously delivered at 7.27 pm; he was born healthy. The second twin, later named Stuart, was born 68 minutes later with severe brain damage; he suffers from cerebral palsy, and is a quadriplegic spastic. Experts at the trial agreed that he should have been born as soon as reasonably practical after his brother and in any event within 20 minutes. Stuart did receive £750 000 compensation (Miles, 1990). The delay in securing the attendance of senior medical staff capable of dealing with the emergency situation was too long and therefore there was a breach of duty. The call system had broken down.

Lord Justice Slade agreed with the submission made by counsel for the appellants and the judge at first instance: that the health authority had to justify the delays if it could under the *res ipsa loquitur* principle. He said:

> 'In my judgement, however, all the most likely explanations for this failure point strongly either (i) to inefficiency in the system for summoning the assistance of the registrar or consultant...or (ii) to negligence by some individual or individuals in the working of that system. This is, in my judgement, accordingly a case where the *res ipsa loquitur* principle had to be applied...([103] 22 BMLR)'

Dillon L.J. did not expressly deal with the desirability of using the principle. Mustill L.J. did not see the case as warranting the application of the principle.

On the issue of *res ipsa loquitur* the case is notable for a number of reasons. The fact that the judges in the case were not united in their view over the application of the principle illustrates the degree of uncertainty that can surround it. Furthermore, the principle was being used in a novel situation: in the organisation of health care services. In practice *res ipsa* is thus only likely to be applicable in exceptional situations.

Who pays the compensation?

The law of tort can be seen as the legal mechanism for the recovery of compensation by the patient. The issue of who is actually responsible for the payment of the compensation is important for nurses. Many worry that if they are negligent that they may be personally liable to pay the patient compensation. Others worry that if their employers pay the compensation to the injured patient their employers may seek to recover the money from them personally. In the NHS damages are paid by the trust, the employer of the negligent nurse.

A number of new schemes and organisations help trusts and health authorities deal with clinical negligence damages claims. These are the Clinical Negligence Scheme for Trusts (CNST), the Existing Liabilities Scheme (ELS) and the National Health Service Litigation Authority (NHSLA). These will be discussed in Chapter 10. They impact directly on nurses involved in negligence cases and generally in the care environment.

Vicarious liability

Employers are liable, along with their employees, for non-authorised acts done in the course of their employment. This principle is known as 'vicarious liability' and it makes the employer jointly and severally liable even when not at fault; it is a form of strict liability. It is a necessary condition that the employees were acting in the course of their employment when they committed the tort and that the action complained of was one which the employee was authorised to undertake. The injured patient can sue the nurse, or both the hospital and the nurse, or just the hospital.

Whatever course is taken, the nurse who committed the negligent act always remains personally responsible and accountable for her or his negligence and it is possible that the employer could seek to recover from the nurse the compensation which has been paid out. However, recent NHS guidance states that attempts should not be made to recover costs from employees in this manner (NHS 1996). The nurse has broken an implied term in the contract of employment that s/he will exercise reasonable care and skill. There is also a statutory provision which would allow the employer to recover any compensation paid out on the negligent nurse's behalf (Civil Liability (Contribution) Act 1978).

Generally speaking, lawyers proceed against the employer and not the employee. If, however, the employer can establish that the nurse was not acting in the course of employment when s/he was negligent, then the lawyers acting for the injured patient could bring an action against the nurse directly. However, in practice such an action is unlikely to go ahead, because it is questionable whether the individual nurse would have the financial resources to pay the compensation. It is not an easy legal task to determine what constitutes action taken in the course of employment. There are many cases on the point and some are quite difficult to reconcile; there is no definitive test.

Direct liability

If a patient was injured, not by the acts or omissions of a nurse, but because of a defect in machinery or because the system of care in the hospital failed, then the hospital could be held directly liable to the injured patient (*Cassidy* v. *Minister of Health* [1951] 1 All ER 574). This is because of what is termed a 'non-delegable duty'. The issue of a health authority or trust's direct liability for medical or nursing negligence is a controversial one. The principle is not clearly recognised by the court but it could have a potentially important effect and impact where an NHS trust contracts out services to an organisation. Where negligence is alleged the injured patient could proceed against the trust, claiming that it was directly liable for the injury which was caused.

Criminal liability and negligent conduct

While in most situations grave carelessness by the nurse will lead to civil proceedings, in some instances a criminal prosecution may result. If a nurse's actions are gravely careless and if death ultimately results then s/he may be prosecuted for manslaughter. While there have been no notable prosecutions of nurses for gross negligence or manslaughter, there have been criminal prosecutions of doctors. In *R* v. *Adomako* ([1994] 3 All ER 79), a patient died after an anaesthetist, during an eye operation, failed to notice that the endotracheal tube assisting the patient's breathing had become disconnected. Evidence at the hearing was to the effect that the conduct of the plaintiff was 'abysmal' with 'gross dereliction of duty'. He was found guilty of manslaughter. Lord MacKay set out in his judgment the basic test for manslaughter in criminal law:

> '...the principles of the law of negligence apply to ascertain whether or not the defendant has been in breach of a duty of care towards the victim who has died. If such a breach of duty has been established the next question is whether that breach of duty caused the death of the victim. If so, the jury must go on to consider whether that breach of duty should be characterised as gross negligence and therefore as a crime. This will depend on the seriousness of the breach of duty committed by the defendant in all the circumstances in which the defendant was placed when it occurred. The jury will have to consider whether the extent to which the defendant's conduct departed from the proper standard of care incumbent upon him, involving as it must have done a risk of death to the patient, was such that it could be judged criminal.'

Application of this test is unlikely to be easy; in effect assessment of what amounts to culpability has been left in the hands of the jury. It is not clear whether the same principles apply to situations in which the defendant has failed to act as those which apply when the defendant has acted. There is a further issue where a nurse makes a mistake and a death of a patient results, but the nurse claims that the negligence results from working in a situation in which there are severe financial constraints and underfunding. Where does liability lie? One possibility is that the trust could be held to be liable on the basis of what is known as 'corporate manslaughter'. This means that the managers are held responsible for the actions of the organisation. (See *R* v. *P&O European Ferries (Dover) Ltd* [1991] 93 Cr App R 72.)

Reform

Concern over the increase in litigation involving health care professionals has led to discussions of alternatives which could be proposed. One approach adopted in Sweden and New Zealand is to enable individuals to claim compensation through a no-fault scheme (Brazier, 1993; McLean, 1993). Under such a scheme they would not have to establish fault by a health professional, merely that the actions of the health professional caused the harm suffered. It appears unlikely that such a scheme would be adopted in this country, at least in the near future. Many are concerned of the costs of such a compensation scheme both in its initial establishment and subsequent operation.

There is a movement towards settling matters without recourse to litigation in this country and at present pilot schemes for 'alternative dispute resolution' are being undertaken by certain health authorities. The aim of an alternative dispute resolution approach is that of encouraging parties to settle without recourse to litigation. The Government also commissioned a major study into the operation of civil litigation by Lord Woolf, who reported in 1996 (Woolf Report, 1996). The implementation of this report will have the consequence of major effects regarding medical negligence litigation. This issue is returned to in Chapter 10.

Conclusions

Nurses do not have to practice to an impeccable standard; only as ordinary skilled nurses would have acted in the circumstances of the case. The legal accountability of the nurse is set by the *Bolam* test. In the next chapter, some specific questions of liability in relation to negligence are considered in the context of various specific issues.

References

Action for Victims of Medical Accidents (1984-85) *Annual Report*. AVMA, London, (i) p. 7.

Barker, K. (1995) 'NHS contracting: shadows in the law of tort.' *Medical Law Review*, **3**, 161.

Brazier, M. (1993) 'The case for a no-fault compensation scheme.' In *Compensation for Damage: An International Perspective* (ed. S. McClean). Aldershot, Dartmouth.

Burton, J. (1993) 'Skin complaint.' *Nursing Times*, **89** (7), 76.

Case histories (1993) 'Delay in diagnosis of retained surgical swab.' *Journal of the Medical Defence Union*, **9**, 6.

Dixon, E. (1984) *The Theatre Nurse and the Law*. Croom Helm, London.

Jones, M.A. (1996) *Medical Negligence*, 2nd edn. Sweet and Maxwell, London.

Jones, M.A. (1996) *Textbook on Torts*, 4th edn. Blackstone Press, London.

Jones, M.A. (1992) 'Medical negligence.' In *Doctors, Patients and the Law* (ed. C. Dyer). Blackwell Scientific Publications, Oxford.

Kennedy, I. and Grubb, A. (1993) 'Commentary, *Bolitho* v. *City and Hackney Health Authority*' (1993). *Med L Rev*, **1**, 241.

Mason, J.K. and McCall Smith, R.A. (1994) *Law and Medical Ethics*, 4th edn. Butterworths, London.

McLean, S. (ed.) (1993) Can no-fault analysis ease the problem of medical injury litigation? In *Compensation for Damage: An International Perspective*, Dartmouth, Aldershot.

Miles, K. (1990) 'Health authority liable for negligent organisation of maternity services - *Bull* v. *Devon Health Authority*.' *AVMA Medical and Legal Journal*, **1**, 11.

Montgomery, J.(1995) 'Negligence.' In *Nursing Law and Ethics* (eds J.H. Tingle and A. Cribb). Blackwell Science, Oxford.

NHS Executive (1996) *NHS Indemnity Arrangements for Clinical Negligence Claims in the NHS.* 96 HR 0024, DOH, Leeds.

Tingle, J.H. (1991) 'First aid law.' *Nursing Times*, **87**, 48.

Tingle, J.H. (1990) 'Eusol and the law.' *Nursing Times*, **86**, 70.

UKCC (1996) *Guidelines for Professional Practice.* United Kingdom Central Council for Nursing, Midwifery and Health Visiting, London.

UKCC (1992) *Code of Professional Conduct.* United Kingdom Central Council for Nursing, Midwifery and Health Visiting, London. (i) clause 3.

Woolf Report (1996) *Access to Justice.* Final Report to the Lord Chancellor on the Civil Justice System in England and Wales. HMSO, London.

Chapter 3

Patient complaints

John Tingle

In many instances when something goes wrong patients are likely to want to know what went wrong, rather than necessarily be concerned to obtain some degree of financial compensation for what has taken place. An effective complaints system has become to be regarded as an essential part of good health care management. More people are complaining than ever before about the care they receive in the NHS. This chapter attempts to explain the complaints procedures in the NHS, in light of recent major changes to the system. At present some uncertainty exists as to how these reforms will operate in practice. It should be noted that the complaint system is separate from the health care professional disciplinary system. (For discussion of the United Kingdom Central Council for Nursing, Midwifery and Health Visiting (UKCC) disciplinary procedures see Chapter 1.) The patient may not be the only person who seeks to complain. Instead, the health professional may want to voice his or her concerns as to the standard of care being provided to patients. Staff complaints are treated separately from patient complaints. This issue is returned to in Chapter 7, where the question of whistleblowing is considered.

Complaints are an inevitable aspect of professional life. Despite the very best intentions and efforts of nursing staff, something will at some time or other go wrong and some patients will always complain. Patients are now much more aware of how to complain, and to whom, and that in appropriate circumstances they can sue. There is evidence of an increase in the number of complaints made about treatment in the NHS. The Health Service Commissioner (HSC) (1996a) quoted figures published by the Department of Health (DOH) showing that 37 350 written complaints were made to NHS bodies in England in 1990-91 and 100 033 in 1994-95. Why has this increase occurred? The rise in complaints may not necessarily be directly attributable to a general deterioration in the quality of the health service, but rather to a much more informed, consumer orientated and less deferential public which maintains high expectations of the health service. A more vocal public is increasingly holding *all* types of professionals to account. There has been a similar increase in the number of complaints received by the ombudsman and in addition initiatives such as the *Patient's Charter* (DOH, 1995a) have helped draw attention to the patient's right to complain. The right is expressed as follows:

> '(To) have any complaint about NHS services (whoever provides them) investigated and to get a quick, full written reply from the chief executive or general manager.'

The media have also increased public awareness of health care complaints by widely reporting cases of medical and nursing negligence. The HSC (1996b) reported high levels of complaints to his office. The Audit Commission (1993) noted an increase in health care complaints:

> 'The number of complaints hospitals receive varies and may depend on where they are (in London and the south-east, hospitals generally receive more complaints than hospitals elsewhere), how big they are, and how well procedures are advertised. But all hospitals throughout the UK report an increase in complaints over the past three years.'

Berrington and Barnwell (1995) discuss the Central Statistical Office publication *Social Trends* (vol. 25) and note:

> 'Britons have become healthier, sometimes wealthier and more likely to own their own homes; higher expectations mean we are also increasingly dissatisfied.'

Health complaints can be seen in a much broader and generalised context; we live now in a much more complaining and litigation conscious society. Health professionals may in some respects be at a disadvantage in that complaints made against them are more likely to attract media attention because of the 'human interest' factor. Finally, where a complaint is made in the context of health care it is not simply a matter of ensuring that a fault is remedied. There is an important issue of public accountability in the context of the NHS (Simanowitz, 1985).

Health care provision is a matter of public funding and of public concern. There is an expectation that health care providers should be accountable. Nurses need to be aware of the complaints process and the fact that they may be the subject of complaints made, whether at informal or formal level. It is also important that the nurse is aware of what rights patients have in this area regarding her or his role as patient advocate.

Complaints and patient confusion

Frequently a patient's complaint may arise from his confusion, anxiety and frustration at not receiving a satisfactory explanation of why something has gone wrong; frustration which may result in anger and trigger off a complaint (Medical Defence Union, 1993). Litigation or a formal complaint might never have taken place had the patient been given an understandable explanation of what had gone wrong and the steps being taken to remedy matters. Vincent, Young and Phillips (1994) surveyed 227 patients and relatives who were taking legal action through five firms of plaintiff solicitors. They found that the decision to take legal action was determined not only by the original injury, but also by insensitive handling and poor communication after the original incident. The following four main factors were identified in the analysis of reasons for litigation:

- Accountability
- Explanation
- Standards of care
- Compensation and admission of negligence.

Patients and relatives wished to see staff disciplined and called to account. They wanted an explanation and felt ignored or neglected after the incident. They also wanted to make sure that the same problem did not happen to anybody else.

Complaints can arise from, what may seem to the health carer, trivial matters. The diabetic clinic may have been very busy and short staffed at a particular time. As a result the patient may have had a long wait for treatment. An overworked nurse may have been a little abrupt when the patient asked how much longer he was going to have to wait. The patient takes offence at what he sees as a personal insult and complains. But some matters are more complex and may raise issues of such gravity that monetary compensation is required as well as an explanation.

Complaints may or may not have a reasonable basis. Truelove (1985) states:

> 'Some people complain only reluctantly and as a last resort, when prompted by a deep emotion. Some complain reasonably on reasonable grounds. Some complain 'unreasonably' on reasonable grounds. Some complain 'reasonably' on unreasonable grounds. A few (usually with a history of psychological disturbance) complain unreasonably on unreasonable grounds. A few seem to be 'born complainants' who relish a battle and will complain on any grounds whatsoever.'

Nevertheless, while some complaints may be unjustifiable it is important that an effective complaints procedure is established and in operation.

Complaint processes in the NHS have changed gradually over the last 10 years. The most significant reform, however, took place on 1 April 1996. New, unified complaint procedures for dealing with complaints about hospitals, community health services and family health services came into effect. The previous procedures were regarded by many as unsatisfactory. As Simanowitz (1995) commented:

> 'If someone of negative intent had sat down to create a system for patients to complain about health care they would have been unlikely to have come up with anything as unhelpful as the present system, if that is what it can be called.'

Different complaints procedures were to be followed depending on where the treatment took place. Each set of procedures had different rules. Fundamentally, there was no common ethos. Not surprisingly, many patients were confused by the complaint procedures.

The Government established a committee to examine the issue. The Wilson Committee report (1994) carefully considered the existing procedures and recommended major reform. The Government response to Wilson, *Acting on Complaints* (DOH, 1995b), was positive and the Wilson Committee recommendation for a two-stage complaints procedure within the NHS, overseen by the HSC (Ombudsman) was accepted. A new simplified procedure, which recognised the NHS patient as a consumer and embodied the principles recommended by the Wilson Committee, came into effect in April 1996. Complaints about hospitals, community health services, and family health services are now dealt with in similar fashion at two clear levels with the HSC sitting at the apex of the complaints system.

Handling complaints

Whatever the complaint, it must be correctly handled. Hospitals should have established standards and protocols on complaint handling. All staff should be aware of these and they should reflect a number of basic principles. Furthermore, the Clinical Negligence Scheme of Trusts (1996) requires by Risk Management Standard No. 6 that an agreed system of managing complaints is in place and that there are a number of areas of assessment. The NHS Training Division (1995) in their *Local Resolution Training Resources Pack* for the NHS Complaints Procedure, states that foundation principles of complaint procedures are those found in the Wilson Committee report (1994), set up by the DOH to review complaints procedures:

- Responsiveness
- Quality enhancement
- Cost effectiveness
- Accessibility
- Impartiality
- Simplicity
- Speed
- Confidentiality
- Accountability

The new complaints procedures should, hopefully, produce a system and culture which helps develop the communication processes between staff and patients, to enable staff to:

Elicit comments in relation to service provision.
Listen to and understand the complaint.
Find out what the complainant wants.
Eliminate adversarial situations.
Acknowledge complainants' feelings.
Be seen to act on matters raised.

These principles will result in improvement in the communication process between patient and health carer which should, in time. work to avoid formal complaints and litigation.

The UKCC (1996), in sections 22 and 23 of their *Guidelines for Professional Practice*, discuss the issue of patient and client communication and recognise that communication is an essential part of good professional practice. A useful communication strategy is outlined, which includes an emphasis on the importance of listening. Hill (1991) of the Medical Defence Union (MDU) also offers some useful guidance on complaint handling:

> 'When dealing with patient's complaints remember the four S's; complaints should be handled SPEEDILY, with SYMPATHY, to the patient's SATISFACTION, and (if indicated) with an expression of SORROW. Conciliation, not confrontation should be the goal.'

It is important to remember that a complaint could result in litigation. Complaints should also be analysed for trends. The success of Risk Management and Quality Assurance strategies is dependent on complaints and claims analysis.

A patient may wish to complain and asks a nurse about appropriate channels. To function effectively as a patient advocate, the nurse must have a reasonable working knowledge and understanding of the complaints system and protocols (Tingle, 1990), in particular her or his own local hospital complaints procedure. Minor complaints can often be handled by the nurse as they arise. More significant complaints should be referred promptly to a line manager.

Guidance issued by the DOH (1996) places great emphasis on resolving complaints as quickly as possible, informally through front line staff, called 'local resolution'. The guidance is not designed to be all-embracing. Individual complaint models can be developed but they must take account of the legal framework, directions and regulations that have been issued.

Local resolution

The trust/health authority must establish a clear local resolution process. According to the DOH guidance, the process should be open, fair, flexible and conciliatory. Its primary purpose should be to give a comprehensive response that satisfies the complainant.

Time limit

There is a time limit on initiating complaints. Normally, a complaint should be made within 6 months from the incident that caused the problem or within 6 months of the date of discovering the problem, provided that this is within 12 months of the incident. There is a discretion to extend this time limit. The complaint can be made orally or in writing, by an existing or former patient or by somebody acting on the patient's behalf.

Complaints manager

A trust/health authority must have a designated complaints manager who oversees the complaints procedure. The manager will receive the complaints from patients and should be readily identifiable to staff and public. If a complaint is not resolved at this informal stage then the complainant can make a request to a convener for an independent review.

Independent review

Trusts/health authorities must appoint at least one person, who may not be one of its own employees, to act in the role of convener. At least one of the persons appointed must be a non-executive of the trust/health authority. There is no automatic right to an independent review of a complaint. A complainant can request an independent review to the convener, either orally or in writing, within 28 calendar days from the completion of the local resolution process. The convener has a discretion to consider requests made outside the time period.

Action by the convener

The convener must obtain from the complainant a signed written statement setting out the complaint and why the complainant is dissatisfied with the investigation of the initial complaint. In deciding whether to convene a panel, the convener would consider a number of factors in consultation with an independent lay chairman from the regional list. Where the complaint concerns a matter of clinical judgement, then clinical advice must be obtained.

Issues which will be examined are whether further action can be taken by the trust or authority towards satisfying the complainant without appointing a panel to investigate the complaint. Alternatively, the trust or health authority may have taken all the action which is practical towards satisfying the complainant, and no further benefit would be achieved by appointing a panel. Although advice must be sought, the decision as whether or not to set up a panel is one ultimately for the convener to make.

Where independent review has been refused, the complainant and any person complained against should be advised of this decision in writing with reasons and whether or not the convener believes there is further action the trust or health authority can take. The complainant must also be advised of his or her right to complain to the HSC. If a panel is to be set up the terms of reference should be stated. If a complainant is dissatisfied following reference back to the trust or health authority, s/he may ask the convener to reconsider whether an independent review panel should be set up.

The panel

The panel consists of three members, one of which, the chairman, is nominated by the Secretary of State. The trust or health authority should also appoint a member to act as convener and there should be a member representative from the purchaser. The panel has discretion over the nature of the procedures to adopt for dealing with the complaint. If there is disagreement as to these procedures then the chairman of the panel has the power to make the ultimate decision. A legally qualified person may accompany a participant and speak to the panel or assessors with the chairman's consent. However, this person must not speak as an advocate for the participant.

Assessors

If the complaint concerns or partly concerns the exercise of clinical judgement then at least two assessors must be appointed. Their role is to advise and make a written report to the panel on matters related to clinical judgement. The assessors are nominated by the Secretary of State from an approved list.

Report of the panel

The report of the panel must include the following matters:

1. Findings of fact relevant to the complaint;
2. Opinion of the panel on the complaint having regard to the findings of fact.
3. Reasons for the panel's opinion.
4. Report of the assessors.
5. Where the panel disagrees with any matter included in the report of the assessors, the reason for its disagreement.

The report may include suggestions which would improve trust or health authority services and the steps that might be taken to satisfy the complainant. It cannot, however, suggest that disciplinary proceedings be taken against any person. The final report will have a restricted circulation and among those who will receive a copy are the complainant, any person named in the complaint, clinical assessors, chairman, chief executives, etc.

End of proceedings

When chief executives receive the reports, they must write to the complainants informing them of any action that is going to be taken or the reasons for taking no action. A complainant's right to apply to the HSC must also be stated

Practice-based complaints procedures

All family health service practitioners (persons undertaking to provide general medical services, general dental services, general ophthalmic services or pharmaceutical services under the National Health Service Act 1977) were required to establish their own practice-based procedures for dealing with patient complaints by 1 April 1996 (NHS Executive, 1996a). The aim of the new system is to try where possible to resolve most complaints at practice level - local resolution. If the complainant does not wish to complain directly to the practice, matters can go to Family Health Services Conciliation. Independent review procedures can be requested where matters remain unresolved.

The complaints procedure is not concerned with practitioner discipline; there is a completely separate and distinct procedure for these matters. The terms of service of GPs and other family health service practitioners have been amended to include the setting up of practice-based complaint systems and the requirement to cooperate with health authority procedures. GPs have discretion in the nature and operation of their practice-based complaints system; however, their system must reflect the national criteria.

National criteria

The criteria include the following:

- Practice-based procedures should be practice owned and managed.
- One person should be nominated to administer the procedure, though how this is done is for the practice to decide.
- Practices must give the procedure publicity and make written information available to anyone who asks for it.
- Complaints should normally be acknowledged within 2 working days;
- An explanation should normally be provided within 10 working days

Guidance is given on a model procedure which includes information on initial contact, the interview, leaflet, acknowledgement, etc. An in-house complaints procedure should be:

- simple and responsive
- accessible and well publicised
- confidential

- understood by all practice staff so that they can advise patients on how to use it
- speedy yet thorough'

A complainant may be unhappy with the outcome of the local practice-based procedure and may request an independent review. Independent review procedures, as discussed above, are applicable to complaints made against GPs. The convener again has responsibility for looking at the complaint in consultation with an independent lay chairperson and deciding whether to agree to a request for independent review. The old formal service committees, as they were known, have gone. It will be recalled that the convener has a number of available options open, which include referring the complaint back to the practice for further consideration (if it appears that the practice-based procedure has not been fully exhausted), or arranging conciliation if it appears that that course would be helpful.

Family health services conciliation

A complainant may not, for some reason, wish to have his or her complaint dealt with by the GP practice complaints procedure. The complainant may not feel it is sufficiently independent. A complainant may also be experiencing difficulties getting the complaint dealt with. In these circumstances the health authority can act as an 'honest broker' and try to resolve the complaint through lay conciliators at local resolution. If the complainant remains dissatisfied then he or she can request an independent review. If a complainant remains dissatisfied after the independent review, or has been denied an independent review, he or she will be able to ask the HSC or Ombudsman to consider investigating the complaint.

Health Service Commissioner (Ombudsman)

The HSC is an official who is independent of the NHS and Government. He is accountable to Parliament for his work. The work of the HSC is overseen by the Select Committee on the Parliamentary Commissioner for Administration. The HSC presents an annual report to both Houses of Parliament and produces periodic volumes of selected investigation reports. The HSC can also issue reports on particular cases or issues. A recent special report was made on investigation of complaint handling by Salford Royal Hospitals NHS Trust (HSC, 1996a) (all these publications are available from HMSO). The HSC now sits at the apex of the complaints system and can investigate complaints about the NHS. The Health Service Commissioner's (Amendment) Act 1996 extended considerably the HSC powers of investigation, which now include the power to investigate matters involving the clinical judgement of health care professionals and to investigate complaints about the family health services provided by GPs, dentists, pharmacists and opticians.

Matters the HSC cannot investigate

The HSC is unable to investigate a number of matters which include:

- Personnel issues such as staff appointments, discipline or pay.
- Complaints about local disciplinary arrangements for family health service providers.
- Commercial or contractual matters unless they relate to services for patients provided under an NHS contract.
- Where the complainant could take legal proceedings. An example would be a clinical negligence claim or a right of appeal reference or review before a tribunal. The HSC can still investigate these matters if satisfied that in the particular circumstances it is not reasonable to expect the complainant to follow this course

Maladministration

The HSC investigates matters where there has been maladministration or failure of service. The HSC and staff subscribe to the following statement of purpose (HSC, 1995):

> 'To investigate impartially and expeditiously complaints about maladministration or failure in service leading to injustice or hardship, and about refusal of access to official information by NHS authorities; to obtain appropriate redress for the complainant; and to promote fairness, integrity and practical improvements in public administration and the quality of service provided to users of the National Health Service.'

What is maladministration?

The term maladministration is a key concept to the understanding of the work and jurisdiction of the HSC. Before a discretionary decision of a trust, health authority or other body or person can be challenged, there must be evidence of maladministration. The term acts as a trigger for the involvement of the HSC. The term is not defined in a statute but is discussed by the HSC (1996a). It includes:

'• Bias
- Neglect
- Inattention
- Delay
- Incompetence
- Ineptitude

- Perversity
- Turpitude
- Arbitrariness
- Rudeness (though that is a matter of degree)
- Unwillingness to treat the complainant as a person with rights
- Refusal to answer reasonable questions
- Neglecting to inform a complainant on request of his or her rights or entitlement
- Knowingly giving advice which is misleading or inadequate
- Ignoring valid advice or overruling considerations which would produce an uncomfortable result for the overruler
- Offering no redress or manifestly disproportionate redress
- Showing bias whether because of colour, sex, or any other grounds
- Omission to notify those who thereby lose a right of appeal
- Refusal to inform adequately of the right of appeal
- Faulty procedures
- Failure by management to monitor compliance with adequate procedures
- Cavalier disregard of guidance which is intended to be followed in the interests of equitable treatment of those who use a service
- Partiality
- Failure to mitigate the effects of rigid adherence to the letter where that produces manifestly in equitable treatment'

The list given is illustrative and not exhaustive. This HSC focus on maladministration does not apply when a complaint relates to a decision taken in the exercise of clinical judgement (HSC, 1996b):

> '...the Ombudsman may uphold the complaint without having regard to considerations of maladministration because the test of maladministration is not apt for clinical decisions.'

The HSC has assessors who are able to advise whether the actions complained of were based on a reasonable and responsible exercise of clinical judgement of a standard which the patient could be reasonably entitled to expect in the circumstances.

Access procedures

Generally speaking, complaints must be made to the HSC by the person directly concerned within 1 year of the matter coming to the person's notice. It is possible that another person or organisation could complain on the patient's behalf. The complaint can even be made after the death of the complainant by the next of kin or some other person or organisation.

The HSC has indicated that he will receive complaints brought by hospital staff on the patient's behalf. The HSC will not normally consider a complaint until the local review stages have been completed. The HSC (Office of HSC, 1996) has provided a special complaint form which can be returned (Appendix 2). Staff employed by NHS bodies, independent providers, family health services practitioners and those working for them can complain to the HSC if they consider that they have suffered hardship or injustice through the complaints procedure operated by trusts/health authorities. Established local grievance procedures must be completed before approaching the HSC.

Investigation

The HSC has staff to assist him in his work; these staff include investigating and screening officers. The HSC also has specialist health care professional advisors in relation to complaints on clinical judgement. The investigation is conducted in private and the procedure is informal. Comments are sought from hospital staff on the complaint. The HSC has the same powers as a High Court judge to obtain information and documents. If staff do not want to cooperate they can be compelled to testify to the HSC. The production of documents and reports can also be formally ordered by the HSC. Relations between the HSC and health authority staff are normally good and these formal measures would only be used as a last resort.

Report

When the investigation is completed the HSC sends a report to the complainant, the relevant NHS authority and to any individual who has had allegations made about him or her in the complaint. The report states whether the complaint or any part of it has been upheld and recommends a remedy. The remedy may take the form of an apology from the health authority and the other parties involved. The HSC report cannot be enforced in a court of law. HSC investigations and findings are separate and quite distinct from court proceedings.

HSC investigations and findings of maladministration have also led the HSC to make detailed recommendations which have included:

- Changes in procedures
- Creation of training programmes
- Improvements in record keeping, etc

The HSC cannot award compensation but does sometimes recommend that an *ex gratia* payment be made to cover a complainant's expenditure or financial loss. An example can be seen in case W.525/91-92. (HSC, 1992c). Damage was caused to the complainant's property by a mentally ill patient jumping naked from a hospital window into the complainant's house. The complainant was dissatisfied with the health authority and hospital's response to the incident. The HSC recommended that the district health authority, as an act of grace, make an *ex gratia* payment without admission of liability to cover the complainant's uninsured loss. The district health authority promised to make a payment to cover half of the complainant's loss.

Errors and failures

HSC reports reveal a wide catalogue of errors and failures which, generally speaking, could have been easily avoided. A large number involve communication failures; the HSC (1992b) commented: '...some topics - such as record keeping, complaints handling and observation of patients - feature regularly in...annual reports'.

Nurses have figured frequently in the reports. In the period 1982/83 until 1991/92, there were 1736 investigations involving nursing (38% of all investigations in this period). Complaints included:

Failure in care
Lack of or incorrect information
Attitudes
Maltreatment (HSC, 1992b).

A useful illustration of the problems, in a nursing context, that can occur can be seen in case W.232/90/91 (HSC, 1992a). A woman was terminally ill with cancer and was also suffering from claustrophobia. She was nursed during the week in a surgical ward and for hospital financial reasons was moved at the weekend to other wards and sometimes a small side room. A decision was eventually made to transfer her to a hospice, where she died 3 days after the transfer. Her husband complained that the weekend ward transfers caused his wife unacceptable distress and that nursing staff in these wards were unaware that his wife suffered from claustrophobia. He said that there had been inadequate nursing care in one ward. He claimed that his wife had not been given help with washing, that pressure sores had been allowed to develop, and her urostomy and ileostomy bags had not been changed regularly. He complained of insensitivity on the part of a ward sister, whom he stated had asked his wife to cut up an incontinence roll when supplies had run out. The roll was inadequate for his wife's needs and he had to buy another one. The sister, he claimed, had also been unwilling to arrange for an ambulance to take his wife to the hospice. Some of the husband's complaints were upheld. The HSC found 'a deplorable lack of regard by management for patient's welfare'. The health authority apologised.

The investigation reports of the HSC provide a useful perspective from which to view the professional accountability of the nurse. The HSC (1995) *Annual Report* contains the following case:

> 'A woman developed a pressure sore while in hospital and I considered that there had been an avoidable delay in taking preventative measures.

I also criticised the poor standard of record keeping. I found that nursing staff had not communicated satisfactorily with the patient's daughter. Board to check that monitoring of pressure area care standards was operating effectively. (S.104/93-94, Tayside HB)'

Complaint handling: The future

We have seen that dramatic and far reaching changes to hospital and general practice complaints systems have taken place. It is perhaps too early to say how well the reforms will go. Criticisms have emerged on a number of matters. The Association of Community Health Councils for England and Wales (ACHCEW, 1996) on local resolution of complaints, argues that to do this requires a revolution in attitudes among NHS staff and that the arrangements for training to bring this about are woefully inadequate. Some other misgivings have been expressed. Harris and Simanowitz (1996) argue that the newly overhauled NHS complaints system lacks true independence from the NHS and places unnecessary restrictions on complainants. They expressed concerns as to the impartiality of the system where a complainant requests an independent review. Requests are screened by a member of the health authority or trust involved. They fear that the HSC, now placed at the apex of the system, will be overloaded with appeals from dissatisfied complainants who have been refused an independent review. They also argue that the 6-month time limit for bringing complaints under the new system is too restrictive. The DOH documentation which has been produced on complaint handling certainly looks very promising, with clear advice on strategies to avoid and handle complaints being given. Much of the success of the new strategy will, however, depend on how well health carers and managers are trained in the underlying philosophy of the system and, realistically, how much time can be devoted to this process.

References

ACHCEW (1996) *CHC Newsletter*, Issue 1, June.

Audit Commission (1993) *What Seems to be the Matter: Communication Between Hospitals and Patients.* HMSO, London.

AVMA (1995) *Medical Accidents.* Action for Victims of Medical Accidents, London, p. 3.

Berrington, L. and Barnwell, R. (1995) 'Britain's moaning minnies who know their rights.' *The Times,* 26 January.

Clinical Negligence Scheme of Trusts (1996) *Risk Management Standards and Procedures: Manual of Guidance.* CNST, Bristol.

Department of Health (1996) *EL 96 (19)* (Executive Letter). *Implementation of New Complaints Procedures: Final Guidance*, 12 March.

Department of Health (1995a) *The Patient's Charter.* DOH, London.

Department of Health (1995b) *Acting On Complaints: The Government Proposals in Response to 'Being Heard', the Report of a Review Committee on NHS Complaints Procedures.* DOH, London.

Harris, T. and Simanowitz, A. (1996) Letter. *The Times*, 13 April.
Health Service Commissioner (1996a) *Investigation of Complaint Handling by Salford Royal Hospital NHS trust*, HMSO, London. *Second Report for Session 1995-96.* HMSO, London.
Health Service Commissioner (1996b) *Annual Report for 1995-96.* HMSO, London.
Health Service Commissioner (1996c) *A Guide to the Work of the Health Service Ombudsman.* Office of HSC, London.
Health Service Commissioner (1995) *Annual Report for 1994-95.* HMSO, London.
Health Service Commissioner (1992a) *Selected Investigations Completed October 1991-March 1992.* HMSO, London.
Health Service Commissioner (1992b) *Annual Report for 1991-92.* HMSO, London.
Health Service Commissioner (1992c) *Selected Investigations Completed, April-September* 1992. HMSO, London.
Hill, G. (1991) *Complaints About Clinical Care: Correct Management*, October. Medical Defence Union, London.
Medical Defence Union (1993) *Talking to Patients*, March. MDU, London.
NHS Executive (1996a) *Practice-Based Complaints Procedures: Guidance for General Practices*, February. NHS Executive.
NHS Executive (1996b) *Complaints, Listening, Acting and Improving: Guidance on Implementation of the NHS Complaints Procedure*, February. NHS Executive, all accompanying EL 96(19).
NHS Training Division (1995) *Local Resolution Training Resources Pack*. NHSE, Leeds.
Office of Health Service Commissioner (1996) *Do You Have a Complaint About the Service You Have Received from the NHS?* Office of HSC, London.
Simanowitz, A. (1995) Patients' complaints in health care provision. In *Nursing Law and Ethics* (eds J.H. Tingle and A. Cribb). Blackwell Science, Oxford.
Simanowitz, A. (1985) 'Standards, Attitudes and Accountability in the Medical Profession.' *Lancet*, 2 (8454) 546.
Tingle, J.H. (1990) 'Complaints and the law.' *Nursing Standard*, **5**(2), 44.
Truelove, A. (1985) 'On handling complaints.' *Hospital and Health Services Review*, September (i) p. 229.
UKCC (1996) *Guidelines for Professional Practice.* United Kingdom Central Council for Nursing, Midwifery and Health Visiting, London.
Vincent C, Young M. and Phillips, A. (1994) 'Why do people sue doctors? A study of patients and relatives taking legal action.' *Lancet*, **343**, 1609.
Wilson Committee Report (1994) *Being Heard, The Report of a Review Committee on NHS Complaints Procedures*, May. DOH, London.

Chapter 4

Legal aspects of expanded role and clinical guidelines and protocols

John Tingle

In the previous chapter the legal obligations of the nurse to exercise care in treating patients were considered. This chapter focuses upon certain specific issues which have important ramifications regarding nursing accountability, such as expanded role, the operation of clinical care guidelines and protocols and nurse prescribing.

Developments in nursing practice

Today the number of tasks undertaken by nurses has increased. This is related to a number of factors, ranging from resource issues such as the need to reduce junior doctors' hours, to the fact that nurses are being entrusted with wider responsibility as a recognition of their role as independent practitioners. Nurses undertake tasks such as ECGs, defibrillation after a heart attack, verification of death (not in cases of unexpected death), taking blood samples, performing male catheterisation (Eaton, 1993). There are nurse-led minor injury units (MIUs) where nurses carry out a variety of activities which can include suturing, X-ray, plaster and refer (Carlisle, 1995). The growth of the nurse's work has been termed 'expanded role' by some commentators. In the past the term 'extended role' was used when discussing the issue of nurses carrying out activities traditionally carried out by doctors (Tingle, 1993.) The position altered, however, in 1992 (DOH 1992). This change followed a report issued by the Standing Medical Advisory Committee and the Standing Nursing and Midwifery Advisory Committee (1989). The United Kingdom Central Council for Nursing, Midwifery and Health Visiting (UKCC) stated that the terms 'extended' or 'extending roles' are no longer favoured as they: '...limit, rather than extend the parameters of practice' (UKCC, 1992a (i)).

The UKCC (1992a) published a document, *The Scope of Professional Practice*, which stated that:

> 'The registered nurse, midwife or health visitor:
> 1. must be satisfied that each aspect of practice is directed to meeting the needs and serving the interests of the patient or client;
> 2. must endeavour always to achieve, maintain and develop knowledge, skill and competence to respond to those needs and interests;
> 3. must honestly acknowledge any limits of personal knowledge and skill and take steps to remedy any relevant deficits in order effectively and appropriately to meet the needs of patients and clients;
> 4. must ensure that any enlargement or adjustment of the scope of personal professional practice must be achieved without compromising or fragmenting existing aspects of professional practice or care and that requirements of the Council's Code of Professional Practice are satisfied through the whole area of practice;
> 5. must recognise and honour the direct or indirect personal accountability borne for all aspects of professional practice; and
> 6. must, in serving the interests of patients and clients and the wider interests of society, avoid inappropriate delegation to others which compromises those interests.'

Many see role expansion as presenting an exciting opportunity to develop new specialisms. However, expanding the nursing role has been controversial and there has been disagreement within the nursing profession as to what approach should be taken. There is no national standard or catalogue of expanded roles. Practices differ from region to region and even within hospitals (Standing Medical Advisory Committee and Standing Nursing and Midwifery Advisory Committee, 1989). The debate is still an intense one. Some nurses argue that nursing may as a result become too technical and less patient centred (Healey, 1996; Giles, 1993; Shepherd, 1993). Eaton (1993) quotes Derek Dean (formerly Director of Policy and Research at the Royal College of Nursing (RCN)):

> 'The worry among nurses, many of whom welcome this additional responsibility, is that they are being asked to do extra work without anyone extra to take the load off them. A lot of members have expressed concern. They have said, "We are being asked to do things and are rushed off our feet".'

Similarly, Waters (1996) quotes RCN community adviser Mark Jones, who presented at a conference a catalogue of cautionary tales illustrating the dangers of nurses overreaching themselves. The list included one case where a practice nurse with no formal midwifery training had taken over antenatal care and had missed a fetus dying *in utero*.

The emphasis today is upon the nurses themselves making the decision as to whether to undertake an expanded role. If the nurse believes that s/he has the necessary competence, then the nurse may undertake the task her- or himself. The UKCC is opposed to the use of certificates of competence. Such certificates state that the nurse has undergone a training programme and thus may be competent to perform a particular task.

> 'In order to bring into proper focus the professional responsibility and consequent accountability of individual practitioners, it is the Council's principles for practice rather than certificates for tasks which should form the basis for adjustments to the scope of practice.(UKCC, 1992a(ii))'

It has been suggested that the fact that a nurse has been given a certificate may give the nurse a false sense of security and lead her or him to think that accountability for actions had shifted to the nurse's assessor. But at the same time, before a nurse undertakes an expanded role, appropriate training is advisable and such knowledge needs to be sustained and updated. The nurse is under a duty to undertake a minimum of five days of study each 3-year period to update her or his knowledge (an activity requirement). A key tool to ensure a safe environment of care may be through the use of guidelines for tasks which have been delegated by doctors to nurses or where a new role has been developed. The issue of guideline development will be discussed later.

It is interesting to note that while the discourse in nursing practice is that of the nurse her- or himself undertaking an expanded role, difficult issues remain as to the boundaries of practice and where ultimate responsibility lies. Nurses may take on an increased role because they are acting as independent practitioners. Alternatively it may be because they have been delegated certain tasks to be performed by doctors. Guidance has been issued by the medical profession on the issue of delegation. The General Medical Council (GMC) (1995) states that:

> '...You may delegate medical care to nurses and other health care staff who are not registered medical practitioners if you believe it is best for the patient. But you must be sure that the person to whom you delegate is competent to undertake the procedure or therapy involved. When delegating care or treatment, you must always pass on enough information about the patient and the treatment needed. You will still be responsible for managing the patient's care.
>
> You must not enable anyone who is not registered with the GMC to carry out tasks that require the knowledge and skills of a doctor.'

Where tasks are delegated, then the doctor delegating the task should follow appropriate guidelines. Should the doctor fail to do so and harm results to the patient, the doctor may be held liable in negligence for the harm caused. It may also be the case that even where the delegation is properly undertaken, the doctor is held ultimately responsible in any event under what is known as the 'captain of the ship' approach (Montgomery, 1992). It is interesting to note that both the GMC and the BMA assume that where delegation takes place, the doctor retains ultimate accountability (BMA, 1996). It may, however, be questioned to what extent such an approach is appropriate as the role of the nurse develops and she is recognised as having greater personal autonomy, and indeed whether the courts would be more likely to hold that the nurse was solely liable where tasks have been legitimately delegated.

The boundaries between tasks which are undertaken as part of expanded role and those which follow from delegation are unclear. Darley and Rumsey (1996) note that the use of language such as delegation is indicative of hierarchy. They suggest that it would be better to talk in terms of 'shared care' or referral; this would have the advantage of emphasising the partnership and teamwork aspects. Martin et al. (1996) suggest that guidance should be drawn up by the professional organisations GMC and UKCC, in conjunction with bodies such as the British Medical Association (BMA) and RCN, regarding such practices. The UKCC in response to feedback from its practitioners is to promote SCOPE and research its impact on clinical practice (Darley and Rumsey, 1996).

Expanded role negligence

Case study

A case involving a negligent practice nurse illustrates some difficulties regarding accountability (Parker and Wilson, 1992):

> A 34-year-old man attended the doctor to have his right ear syringed. On examination the GP suspected that he had an abscess and prescribed penicillin and asked him to return in one week to see the nurse and have his ear syringed. When the patient returned his ear was syringed by a locum practice nurse and the patient later admitted that during the procedure he had felt excruciating pain and dizziness...He returned to the surgery complaining of a sore ear and the nurse referred him to the doctor. On examination he was found to have a perforated eardrum...he made a good recovery but sued alleging negligence...the GP was found to have fallen below the acceptable standard of care in delegating the procedure to the nurse without first having established her competence. The nurse had not performed ear syringing for some 20 years. The Medical Defence Union (MDU) settled the claim.

Medical negligence and professional misconduct

The crucial issue for the employer then is to ensure that, first of all, the nurse is lawfully undertaking the task. The GP in the case above should have at least asked the nurse whether she had performed an ear syringe before and, if so, how long ago. On the facts of the case, the GP could be viewed as wrongfully assigning the procedure to the practice nurse. This may mean that the GP was acting negligently. Can the present system deal with the nurse who feels that s/he will 'have a go' at an expanded role, taking a very liberal view of her or his own competence and experience? Last et al. (1992) raise the same point:

> 'How can chief nurses, directors of nursing services and nurse managers be sure that all practitioners are safe to enlarge the scope of their practice? How can managers allow those who are able to fly to do so, yet provide a safety net to those who could never fly, or even worse, those who think they can but cannot, from falling down?'

Managers, doctors and nurses have to be trusted to operate the system satisfactorily and in a way which does not compromise patient safety. Overloading the nurse may also have implications for the management should the nurse be unable to perform her or his role because s/he has developed some form of stress-related illness. This issue is returned to in the section on stress at work in Chapter 9.

Legal standard of care to be exercised by a nurse performing an expanded role

Where a nurse performs traditional nursing duties the standard of practice required is that of the ordinary skilled nurse in her or his speciality in the circumstances of the case - the *Bolam* principle. But what is the standard of care s/he must reach if performing an expanded role? Guidance can be taken from the case *Wilsher* v. *Essex Area Health Authority* ([1986] 3 All ER 801).

Wilsher case

The plaintiff, Martin Wilsher, was an infant child born about 3 months early. He was very ill. He was placed in a special care baby unit where a junior and inexperienced doctor monitoring the oxygen in the plaintiff's bloodstream made a mistake and mistakenly inserted a catheter into a vein rather than an artery. He asked a senior doctor to check what he had done. The registrar failed to notice the mistake, and when replacing the catheter himself some hours later made the same mistake himself. The catheter monitor failed to register correctly the amount of oxygen in the baby's bloodstream. He was given excess oxygen. It was alleged that the excess oxygen in his bloodstream had caused an incurable condition of the retina, retrolental fibroplasia. Martin is now completely blind. A key issue discussed by the Court of Appeal was the standard of legal care to be exercised by the junior doctor in the case. Mustill L.J. stated:

> 'In a case such as the present, the standard is not just that of the averagely competent and well-informed junior houseman (or whatever

the position of the doctor) but of such a person who fills a post in a unit offering a highly specialised service.' (at p 813)

Glidewell L.J. stated:

'In my view, the law requires the trainee or learner to be judged by the same standard as his more experienced colleagues. If it did not, inexperience would frequently be urged as a defence to an action for professional negligence. (p. 831)'

On the facts before the court the junior doctor was not found negligent. He had done the reasonable thing and asked his superior, but the registrar was found to be negligent. The case went on appeal to the House of Lords on the issue of causation and eventually was set down for retrial. The case was settled for £116 724.40 (Kerry, 1991). (This case is quoted by the UKCC (1996) in Section 16 of their *Guidelines* in Appendix 1.) The key point to be taken from the *Wilsher* case is that a nurse is liable to be judged by the professional standard of the post which s/he is performing at that time. This means that if the nurse is performing an expanded role, s/he is expected to operate at the level of skill and competence outlined in the expanded role. A further point is that, as Kloss (1988) argues:

'If a nurse undertakes a task for which she knows she has insufficient training, this in itself may constitute negligence, even if she is acting on the orders of a doctor... If a nurse takes on the doctor's role she will be judged by the standard of the reasonable doctor.'

There is much older legal authority (*Philips* v. *William Whitley Ltd* (1938)) ([1958] All ER 560) which could be used to argue against the *Wilsher* elevated legal standard of care proposition. It appears that the *Wilsher* approach is more likely to be followed. The recent case of *Djemal* v. *Bexley Health Authority* [1995] 6 Med LR 269 supports the *Wilsher* approach.

The issue of the appropriate standard of legal care for nurses performing medical tasks to exercise has been brought into sharp focus by a number of recent initiatives where new health care professional posts have been created which involve the performance of some medical activities for example, transplant clinician's assistants and cardiac surgeons' assistants. These posts can be occupied by nurses or other health care professionals. If a negligence case involving one of these staff occurred, the court would have difficulty in assessing the appropriate standard of care for the professional to exercise. The posts are so new and there may only be one or two in existence. The court could look at the nature of the tasks performed and determine who normally performs those tasks. If doctors normally undertake them then a medical standard of care and skill will be expected (Naish, 1995; Peysner, 1995; Caine, 1993). Dowling et al. (1996) highlight some useful criteria that a court considering an expanded role case might take into account in determining the standard of care. These include the nature of the task and the way the nurse 'holds her/himself out' to patients. With regard to the second of these criteria, relevant factors would include dress, name badge, language, socialisation and the way the nurse is perceived by patients.

Conclusions

If the nurse undertakes a role previously undertaken by a medical practitioner then her or his competence to perform that role is that of the level of the medical practitioner. The courts may be looking for the nurse to exercise and maintain medical knowledge, and if the nurse cannot demonstrate this s/he could be found negligent and in breach of the UKCC Professional Code of Conduct (UKCC, 1992b). Inexperience is not a defence to a nursing negligence action. It is very important that nursing staff closely adhere to the UKCC (1992a) *Scope of Professional Practice principles*, particularly principle 9:3, which relates to taking steps to remedy deficits in knowledge.

Advanced practice situations

Clinical guidelines, protocols and the law

The setting of guidelines or protocols is fast becoming an increasingly important aspect of nursing and health care as strategies to ensure quality and avoid risk take effect. These tools broadly set out the procedure to be followed by the nurse in an advanced practice situation, for example the MIU or the Well Women clinic. A GP may develop, with the practice nurse, a guideline or a protocol for the giving of inoculations. The practice of setting guidelines or protocols raises important professional and legal issues. It should be noted at the outset, however, that the use of terminology by authors in the literature is not consistent or clear. As well as clinical guidelines or protocols, a variety of other terms such as practice parameters, clinical pathways, and algorithms are used, often to describe the same tool.

Guidelines or protocols can be seen to be guidance statements based on sound practice. For ease of reference, the term clinical guidelines will be used. The DOH (1996a) defines clinical guidelines as 'systematically developed statements which assist the individual clinician and patient in making decisions about appropriate health care for specific conditions'.

Legal issues

Clinical guidelines raise a number of important legal issues. Fundamentally, the existence of clinical guidelines may impact upon the operation of the *Bolam* test (see Chapter 2). If a guideline is in existence and a nurse has failed to follow it, then this may be a factor which a court takes into consideration when discussing the scope of professional accountability. Nonetheless the fact that a guideline exists does not mean that the court will accept the guideline. As noted in the previous chapter, the court may overrule the decision of a responsible body of professional practice.

Reasonable clinical guidelines

The *Bolam* principle will apply to the creation and use of clinical guidelines. The case of *Early* v. *Newham Health Authority* ([1994] 5 Med LR 214) illustrates the application of the case to clinical guidelines:

Early case
The plaintiff, aged 13 years, was having an appendectomy. The anaesthetist gave an intravenous injection of thiopentone (100 g phentonyl and 100 mg of suxamethonium). Unfortunately he was unable to successfully intubate the plaintiff. The effect of the thiopentone wore off before the effect of the short-term paralysing drug, suxamethonium, wore off and the plaintiff came to. She came to in a state of panic and distress as she was still partly paralysed by the drug. She alleged that the anaesthetist was negligent in failing to intubate her the first time and that the health authority's failed intubation guidelines were faulty. No negligence was found.

The judge considered the guidelines and found them reasonable. He was not satisfied that the guidelines were such that no reasonably competent authority would have adopted them. Before the hospital had adopted the guidelines they were put before the Division of Anaesthesia and the consultants discussed them. They decided that this was the proper procedure to adopt and minutes of the discussion were kept. The key point was that the judge found that a responsible body of medical opinion in the *Bolam* sense would have adopted the failed intubation guidelines that were used. The standard of legal care was therefore satisfied in the case.

In order to satisfy the legal standard of care under *Bolam*, nurses, in drafting and using clinical guidelines, have to act as ordinary skilled nurses in their speciality would have acted. There must be a responsible body of opinion, albeit minority opinion, which regards their practice as proper.

Inappropriate use of clinical guidelines

Situations change and a clinical guidelines drafted some months previously may not now fit into the appropriate clinical care setting. Resource levels may have deteriorated or there may have been staffing changes affecting the ward skill mix. The conventional wisdom on a ward may be that a particular clinical guideline is no longer appropriate. If there are reasonable concerns about the effectiveness and safety of a clinical guideline then good practice dictates that it should be withdrawn and re-evaluated. It may be negligent not to do so as, noted in Chapter 2, health care professionals are required to keep up to date as to the scope of their professional practice.

Not a substitute for professional judgement

When using clinical guidelines, nurses must always practice as reflective practitioners and responsibly exercise their clinical discretion. They must use their own professional judgement and skill and judge the appropriateness of the clinical guidelines for the particular care situation. If they decide to deviate from a clinical guideline then they should record on the notes their reasons for so doing. If unsure about the use of a clinical guideline then advice should be sought from more experienced colleagues.

Clinical guidelines should be reviewed systematically

If a particular clinical guideline became an issue in a nursing negligence case, a key issue would be the review system in operation in the hospital or surgery. The court would want to be satisfied that a clinical guideline was being used appropriately and updated where necessary. Concepts of risk management and quality assurance would also demand a systematic review system.

Clinical guidelines are legally discoverable

Clinical guidelines which were used in the care of a patient would be relevant documents for the purposes of a nursing negligence action. The clinical guideline would be subject to a fairly detailed examination in court. Having a clinical guideline based on reasonable criteria, good research and good practice would provide an indication that a reasonable and reflective care system is in operation. The key point would be to show that the clinical guideline was appropriate to the circumstances of the particular case and was followed by the staff involved. The fact that it was followed or not followed should always be recorded. A clinical guideline shows at the very least that there is a *controlled* environment of care.

Evidence based clinical guidelines

There has been a development of what is known as evidence based medicine and nursing. While this is controversial, it is certainly the case that if a particular approach was deemed to be appropriate after an evidence based evaluation had taken place, then this may be held to be accepted professional practice. Again, however, that does not mean that there would be automatic judicial acceptance. A court examining a clinical guideline would be looking at the information which underpins the clinical guideline, quality of research and clinical practice. Unrealistic clinical guidelines which tried to do too much and those based on poor research, practice, etc. would be criticised by the NHS Executive (DOH, 1996a).

Conclusions

Clinical guidelines do raise a number of important legal issues. They are being used in legal proceedings and will be seen increasingly as an established quality improvement and clinical risk management tool in the health care environment. Clinical guidelines must be used reflectively. They are not substitutes for professional judgement. Effectively used, they have the potential to reduce the level of complaints and litigation in health care by improving communication processes and the quality of care.

Nurse prescribing

One way in which the role of the nurse appears set to develop in the future is the nurse having a wider role in prescribing drugs/medical appliances. In 1986 the Cumberlege report stated that community nurses should have prescribing rights. This was followed by a Crown Report in 1989 which stated that health visitors and nurses should have the power to prescribe medication from a 'nurse's formulary' to benefit patients. Legislation was introduced in 1992 in the form of the Medicinal Products (Prescription by Nurses) Act of that year. At present, nurse prescribing is being undertaken in the form of a number of pilot studies, eight sites in England and two in Scotland. The Government announced in February 1997 that the pilot was to be extended to a further 1200 nurses in 10 trusts. This is a different procedure from a situation in which a nurse administers a drug under a protocol, as in this situation it is the *doctor* who has responsibility for the prescribing. They must prescribe as in accordance with the *Nurse Prescriber's Formulary*. Items included are dressings, appliances, paracetamol and carbaryl.

A Midwives Supply Order allows midwives to possess and use certain controlled drugs. Powers also have been given to enable occupational health nurses to administer prescription only drugs. This may be undertaken as long as they do so only in writing and under a doctor's supervision (Medicines (Products Other Than Veterinary Drugs)(Prescription Only) Order 1983 SI 1983 No. 1212 as amended; NHS Pharmaceutical Services(Amendment) Regulations SI 1996 No. 698 r8).

Nurses have also been administering medication in accordance with protocols produced by doctors, who themselves would actually prescribe the drug. Controversy arose in 1996 over this practice. Advice was given by union lawyers to the effect that this was illegal (Naish and Garbett, 1996). In contrast, the MDU stated that nurses could administer such medication as long as they were working to a protocol. This, it is argued, is in accordance with section 58(2)(b) Medicines Act 1968 which provides that:

> 'No person shall administer (otherwise than to himself) any such medicinal product unless he is an appropriate practitioner or a person acting in accordance with the directions of an appropriate practitioner.'

The appropriate practitioner would be the doctor in this instance. The arguments advanced by the MDU are in accordance with the guidance issued by the UKCC to the effect that:

> 'Nurses can administer medicines according to the directions of a doctor and a detailed protocol would satisfy this requirement. However, nurses cannot supply medicines for the patient to take away unless there is a signed prescription.'

Nonetheless, there is one question mark regarding the status of administration under protocol (Mayor, 1997). It appears that the direction under the statute applies to a specified individual and it has been argued that this would not cover administration to groups of patients. The whole issue of nurse prescribing is now the subject of a review by the Department of Health, to be chaired by Dr June Crown (DOH, 1996b). This will be undertaken over 12 months. Its purpose is to:

> 'develop a consistent framework to determine in what circumstances health professionals could undertake new roles with regard to the prescribing, administration or supply of medicines in the course of clinical practice; and to consider possible implications for legislation, and for professional training and standards.'

Legislation in this area is eagerly awaited to alleviate the uncertainties.

Where nurses act as prescribers they must ensure that they are acting within the powers given by statute. When prescribing drugs the nurse will be judged by the standard of the experienced nurse undertaking such a role. If nurses are involved in prescribing drugs, then they must check the dose given; negligent prescription of an overdose may lead to an action in negligence (*Dwyer* v. *Roderick* (1983) 127 SJ 806) as may writing an illegible prescription (*Prendergast* v. *Sam and Dee; The Times*, [1989] and 1 Med LR 36).

Developments in nursing practice may thus result in the increased possibility of litigation. Practical aspects of the litigation process are considered in Chapter 10.

References

BMA (1996) *Joint Consultants Committee Proptecting Patient Safety* BMA 1996.

Caine, N. (1993) 'Heart to heart.' *Health Service Journal*, **103**(5370), 22.

Carlisle, D. (1995) 'Nurse-led unity.' *Nursing Times*, **91**(47),14.

Darley, M. and Rumsey, M. (1996) The scope of professional practice: work to date. *Nursing Times*, 11(4), 32.

Department of Health (1996a) *Promoting Clinical Effectiveness: A Framework for Action in and Through the NHS*. DOH, London.

Department of Health (1996b) *Delivering the Future*. DOH, London.

Department of Health (1992) PL/CNO (92)4, The extended role of the nurse. *Scope of Professional Practice*, 19 June. DOH, London.

Dowling, S., Martin, R., Skidmore, P., Doyal, L., Cameron, A. and Lloyd, S. (1996) 'Nurses taking on junior doctor's work: a confusion of accountability.' *British Medical Journal*, *312*, 1211-14.

Eaton, L. (1993) 'Vein hopes.' *Nursing Times*, **89**(36), 18.

General Medical Council (1995) *Duties of a Doctor: Guidance from the General Medical Council, Good Medical Practice*. GMC, London, p. 9.

Giles, S. (1993) 'Passing the buck.' *Nursing Times*, **89**(28), 42.

Healy, P. (1996) 'Nurses doing junior doctor's work are safe claims unions.' *Nursing Standard*, **10**(34), 5.

Kerry, D.G. (1991) 'Lawyers comment, *Martin Wilsher* v. *Essex Area Health Authority* and Causation.' *AVMA Medical Legal Journal*, 12.

Kloss, D.K. (1988) Demarcation in medical practice: the extended role of the nurse. *Professional Negligence*, **4**(2), 41.

Last, T., Seld, N., Kassat, J. and Rawan, A. (1992) 'Extended role of the nurse in ICU.' *British Journal of Nursing*, **1**(13), 675.

Mayor, S. (1997) 'Working to protocol.' *Practice Nurse*, **13**(4), 187.

Montgomery, J. (1992) Doctors handmaidens: the legal contribution. In (S. McVeigh and S. Whelar, eds), *Law Health and Medical Regulation*. Dartmouth, Aldershot.

Naish, J. (1995) 'The extended role of the nurse: risk management implications.' *Health Care Risk Report,* **1**, 22-24.

Naish, J. and Garbett, R. (1996) 'Don't administer drugs, says union.' *Nursing Times*, **92**(47), 5.

Parker, S. and Wilson, C. (1992) *An Introduction to Medico-Legal Aspects of Practice Nursing*. MDU, London.

Peysner, J. (1995) 'The captain on the bridge.' *Health Care Risk Report*, **1**, 8.

Shepherd, J. (1993) 'Nurses are changing not extending their roles.' *British Journal of Nursing*, **2**,(9), 447.

Standing Medical Advisory Committee and the Standing Nursing and Midwifery Advisory Committee Joint Working Party on Extended Role (1989) DHSS Professional Letter, PL/CMO, (89), 7.

Tingle, J.H. (1993) 'The extended role of the nurse; legal implications.' *Care of the Critically Ill*, **9**(1), 30-34.

UKCC (1996) *Guidelines for Professional Practice.* United Kingdom Central Council for Nursing, Midwifery and Health Visiting, London.

UKCC (1992a) *The Scope of Professional Practice.* United Kingdom Central Council for Nursing, Midwifery and Health Visiting, London, (i) p. 7; (ii) p. 8.

UKCC (1992b) *Code of Professional Conduct.* United Kingdom Central Council for Nursing, Midwifery and Health Visiting, London.

UKCC (1992c) *Standards for the Administration of Medicines.* United Kingdom Central Council for Nursing, Midwifery and Health Visiting, London.

Waters, J. (1996) 'Horror stories warn of need for training.' *Nursing Times*, **92**(16), 9.

Chapter 5

Consent to treatment I: General principles

Jean McHale

One of the most fundamental principles of health care law and ethics is that treatment should be given only with the patient's consent. The nurse is frequently the person who has to obtain the patient's consent to treatment, whether on the wards or in the community. Even if the doctor has the task of obtaining the patient's consent, the patient may turn to the nurse for clarification or further information regarding the proposed treatment. This chapter begins by considering the types of consent: express and implied, written and oral. Considered secondly is when a patient is legally capable of giving consent and the basis on which treatment may be given to an incompetent patient. Third, liability in criminal and civil law is discussed where treatment is given without consent.

Types of consent

Consent forms

Nurses are familiar with the consent forms given to patients to sign before they go in for an operation. The Department of Health (1992) has published model consent forms which provide guidance to health professionals. In law, while a consent form may provide evidence that the patient has consented, the act of signing a form does not itself make the consent legally valid. What is important is that the consent which is given is 'real', that is to say it has been obtained freely, without pressure being placed upon the patient and that the patient understands the implications of what s/he is consenting to. There may be situations in which consent may be implied through the patient's actions. But considered consent is necessary in relation to all serious medical procedures, and failure to obtain that consent may leave a nurse in danger of being held liable in the criminal courts, or of being sued for damages in the civil courts.

Express and implied consent

Consent may be either express or implied. Consent may be expressly given in writing or orally. Alternatively, a patient may through her actions signify consent, for example the patient proffering her wrist to be bandaged. There are risks in assuming that a patient, in seeking treatment, is consenting to any medical procedure being undertaken. There has been much discussion as to whether, when blood is taken from a patient, it is necessary to obtain the patient's consent for undertaking tests on each individual sample. Particular difficulties have arisen if it is proposed to test one of the samples to determine a patient's HIV status. The simple fact that an HIV test has been undertaken may have considerable repercussions for the patient regarding employment and insurance. The United Kingdom Central Council for Nursing, Midwifery and Health Visiting (UKCC) has issued guidance which states that if a nurse takes blood from a patient without that patient's consent or s/he cooperates in blood being removed without the patient's consent, the nurse may be reported to the UKCC for misconduct (UKCC, 1993i). They do, however, recognise that in certain 'rare and exceptional circumstances' blood may be tested without the patient's consent (UKCC, 1993ii). The guidance does not explain what these circumstances may be; they possibly could include the fact that in the future a cure may be found, and thus to test might facilitate diagnosis and treatment.

Capacity

Generally patients are presumed capable of making their own treatment decisions. But in some situations capacity may be called into question. A patient may not appear to understand what he has been told or may appear confused. The nurse may need to assess whether this patient is capable of making a particular treatment decision. This task may prove to be particularly difficult if a person is mentally handicapped or suffers from fluctuating mental capacity. In *Re C* the court upheld the right of a 68-year-old paranoid schizophrenic who had developed gangrene in his foot to prevent amputation in the future without his express written consent (*Re C* [1994] All ER 819). Thorpe J. suggested a three part test to determine whether a patient possessed capacity. Did the patient comprehend the information given to him or her? Did s/he believe it? Had s/he weighed up the information balancing needs and risks before reaching a decision? At the hearing it was claimed that C was not competent because of his delusions that he was a doctor, and that whatever treatment was given to him was calculated to destroy his body. But despite these claims Thorpe J. held that he was satisfied that C was capable of giving consent because he understood and had retained the relevant treatment information and believed it and had arrived at a clear choice. One difficulty with the test laid down in *Re C* is that it makes capacity dependent upon the information which the patient is actually given (Grubb, 1994). If the nurse provides a patient with a great deal of complex information, the patient may not understand it and so it may not fall within the definition of capacity set out in *Re C*, whereas had the patient been given a very simple basic explanation about the same treatment procedure s/he would have possessed the necessary capacity to consent.

Some guidance to health care professionals as to how to approach the assessment of capacity is contained in a document produced by the British Medical Association in conjunction with the Law Society (the solicitors' professional organisation) and this provides a useful source of reference for the nurse (BMA/Law Society, 1996). They suggest that a decision about capacity should be made on the basis of full information. The health professional should have access to all past medical/psychiatric records. Where appropriate, assessments should be obtained from a clinical psychologist, nurse or social worker. They note that information from relatives and carers is important, although needs to be approached with caution. The guidelines state that views of relatives/carers:

> '...may give clues as to whether current behaviour and thinking reflects an abnormal mental state. Aspects of a person's current thinking may derive not from a medical disability but from a normal personality, or from a particular cultural or ethical background and this may be of great importance in determining capacity. It may even be necessary for the doctor to seek advice from others on such cultural issues, or to suggest that the patient be examined by a doctor of a cultural or ethical background similar to the person being assessed.'

These are useful guidelines and should provide a reference point for the nurse when involved in the consent process. Some very difficult and sensitive issues arise where treatment is refused on ethical/religious grounds. Certain ramifications of these issues are explored in the context of treatment refusal below.

The Law Commission, a body established by the Government to examine areas of law and make recommendations for reform, undertook a study involving treatment of the mentally incompetent and published its recommendations in its report *Mental Incapacity* (Law Commission, 1995). It recommended that capacity to make decisions should be assessed on the balance of probabilities (Law Commission, 1995i). As with the test suggested by Thorpe J. in *ReC*, any test for capacity should be *decision specific*; this emphasises the fact that a person may be capable of making one decision while at the same time being incapable of making another decision. It proposed that legislation should provide that a person should be deemed to lack capacity if at the material time s/he is:

'1. unable by reason of mental disability to make a decision on the matter in question, or

2. unable to communicate a decision on that matter because s/he is unconscious or for any other reason.'

Mental disability was defined by the Law Commission (1995ii) as being:

> 'any disability or disorder of the mind or brain, whether permanent or temporary, which results in an impairment or disturbance of mental functioning.'

The Law Commission (1995 iii) recommended that a person should be unable to make a decision on the basis of mental disability,

> '...if the disability is such that, at the time when the decision needs to be made he or she is unable to understand or to retain the information relevant to the decision, including information about the reasonably foreseeable consequences of failing to make that decision.'

It suggested that a person who, while s/he understands the information given is not able to absorb it, should be held to lack capacity. An example of such a situation is that of a person suffering from a compulsive disorder. The Law Commission (1995iv) recommended that the patient show a basic level of comprehension of the information given 'in broad terms and simple language'. There is a danger that a person is believed to lack capacity when in fact it is not that the person is unable to make a decision, but that there are problems both in communicating information and in receiving that information. The Law Commission noted this difficulty and suggested that, wherever possible, specialists in communication skills should be used. The Law Commission also recommended that the Secretary of State should prepare a code of practice for guidance in such decision making. The contents of any such code would be of vital importance in respecting patient autonomy. It seems that these proposals in this form are now unlikely to become law. In January 1996 the Lord Chancellor indicated that the Government was instead intending to issue its own consultation document (Lord Chancellor's Department, 1996).

Should capacity include the right to make an 'irrational' decision?

If a patient refuses treatment on what the nurse treating him or her regards as an irrational basis, can treatment still be given? As Brazier (1991) comments, an elderly woman with a diseased tooth may have sufficient capacity to understand the suggestion made to her that it should be removed, but she may nevertheless allow her fear of dentists and of the pain of treatment to overcome her wish to have the tooth extracted. One approach to problem patients such as this elderly lady would be to categorise her decision as 'irrational' and to override her decision. A variation on this approach suggested by Kennedy (1991) is that an irrational decision should be respected where it derives from long-held beliefs and values on the basis of which a patient has run his or her life, but not if it is the result of a temporary delusion. Nevertheless, attempting to distinguish between different 'irrational' decisions may be difficult practically. Furthermore, there is also a real risk that those refusals which are found to be 'irrational' will be those of the mentally handicapped and the demented patient (Brazier, 1991).

Fluctuating capacity

An elderly lady is cared for in a nursing home. She has good days and bad days. She can throw tantrums and yet later appear totally lucid. How far do the nurses caring for her need to respect her wishes? Where a patient has a fluctuating mental state it may be acutely difficult to assess capacity and create real difficulties for the nurses treating the patient. In such a situation it is tempting to say she lacks capacity, because English law allows a mentally incompetent patient to be given such treatment as those treating her believe to be in her best interests (*Re F* [1990] 1 AC 1). In *Re T* ([1992] 4 All ER 649) the Court of Appeal held that the capacity of an adult patient is to be judged by reference to the particular decision to be made. This approach was at variance with an earlier Court of Appeal decision in which it was held that a child with fluctuating mental capacity was to be regarded as totally incapable (*Re R* [1991] 4 All ER 177). The approach in *Re T* is surely right, reinforced by the decision in *Re C* which states that the test for capacity is decision specific.

The BMA and the Law Society in their guidelines (BMA/Law Society 1996) provide a number of suggestions for dealing with patients with fluctuating capacity:

'• Any treatable medical condition which affects capacity should be treated before a final assessment is made.
- Incapacity may be temporary albeit for a prolonged period. For example, an older patient with an acute confusional state caused by infection may continue to improve for some time after successful treatment. If a person's condition is likely to improve, the assessment of capacity, should, if possible, be delayed.
- Some conditions, for example dementia, may give rise to fluctuating capacity. Thus, although a person with dementia may lack capacity at the time of one assessment, the result may be different if a second assessment is undertaken during a lucid interval. In cases of fluctuating capacity the medical report should detail the level of capacity during periods of maximal and minimal disability.'

In assessing capacity, in practice much will depend upon the discretion of the individual practitioner. In making the decision, the nurse should keep in mind clause 5 of the UKCC Code, which requires her or him to:

> 'work in an open and cooperative manner with patients, clients and their families, foster their independence and recognise and respect their involvement in the planning and delivery of care.'

Good practice would suggest that as far as possible patients should be left to make their own decisions.

The mentally incompetent patient

Best interest test

Take a situation in which a nurse is asked to care for a patient who has profound mental handicap, or severe brain damage: on what basis can s/he lawfully treat that patient? Until 1990, the legal position as to treating mentally incompetent adult patients was uncertain. Prior to the Mental Health Act 1983 the court had had an 'inherent jurisdiction' to act for the benefit of incompetent adult patients, as they have today with regard to child patients (see Chapter 6). The basis for such treatment was discussed by the House of Lords in 1990. In *Re F* ([1990] AC 1), the court was asked to authorise the sterilisation of a 36-year-old mentally handicapped woman. The House of Lords held that the operation could be undertaken; it held that the court had no power to authorise treatment of a mentally incompetent adult through the use of inherent jurisdiction as it had regarding a child patient (see Chapter 6). Prior to *Re F* it was common practice to get the relatives to sign the consent form. In *Re F* the court said that such consent had no legal effect. No one had a legal right to give consent on behalf of a mentally incompetent adult. However, that did not mean that treatment could not be given. The House of Lords said treatment could be given on the grounds of necessity where this was in the patient's best interests.

'Best interests' is assessed by reference to what a responsible body of professional practice would regard as being in this patient's best interests (the *Bolam* test discussed in Chapter 2). The basis for the 'best interests' test in *Re F* has been criticised. For example, it has been suggested that the test raises questions of value and social policy, issues which are not the sole preserve of doctors (Kennedy and Grubb, 1994). The nurse acting as the patient's advocate may take the view that what a doctor believes to be medically expedient is not actually in that patient's best interests. The nurse should be able to raise concerns and to take the matter further should s/he believe that the patient's interests are being disregarded.

What medical procedures are capable of being authorised under the 'best interests' principle was left uncertain after *Re F*. While it appears that generally therapeutic procedures would clearly fall within 'best interests', the legality of many non-therapeutic procedures such as non-therapeutic clinical trials is questionable. This issue is returned to below.

The Law Commission proposed reform of the 'best interests' test (Law Commission: 1995v). They recommended a set of criteria to be taken into account in determining 'best interests'. These are:

'(1) ascertainable past and present wishes and feelings of the person concerned and the factors that a person would consider if unable to do so;

(2) the need to permit and encourage the person to participate or to improve his or her ability to participate as fully as possible in anything done for and any decision affecting him or her;
(3) the views of other people whom it is appropriate and practicable to consult about the person's wishes and feelings and what would be in his or her best interests;
(4) whether the purpose for which any action or decision is required can be as effectively achieved in a manner less restrictive of the person's freedom of action.'

Such an approach could facilitate decision making. Nevertheless, there may be practical problems in the application of such a test. How would it operate, and how would the relevant criteria be weighed against each other? The Law Commission (1995vi) recommended that an appropriate approach would be the development of a code of practice to facilitate health professionals in ascertaining best interests.

In *Re F* the court said that there was no legal duty to refer all cases concerning treatment of a mentally incompetent adult to the court for approval. Nevertheless in certain situations as, for example, before major surgery is performed, it believed that referral of the issue to the court would be desirable. This raises the question of whether it is appropriate to leave this assessment to the health professional at all. The Law Commission, in its report (1995), suggested that the decision to undertake certain clinical procedures upon mentally incompetent adults should be referred to a decision maker outside those immediately caring for the patient. In some situations, the Commission suggested, the decision should be subject to a second opinion. Cases involving authorisation of serious treatment may be referred to a new body, called a 'judicial forum', a court with specialist expertise in such treatment issues.

Procedures ancillary to treatment

There are a number of practical difficulties in treating mentally incompetent adults. Treatment can be given regardless of consent if it can be shown to be in the patient's best interests. But the patient cannot be confined to one particular place while treatment is provided, unless certain statutory powers such as those under the Mental Health Act 1983 apply. Frequently a confused elderly person may be placed in a bed which has cot sides to stop him or her from falling out. But is this justifiable? Is it part of treatment? It might be argued that to restrain the patient in this situation might even constitute the tort of false imprisonment. The powers of treatment of such patients urgently require clarification.

Criminal law liability

Bringing a criminal law prosecution against a nurse or doctor where a medical procedure has been undertaken without consent may seem only a remote possibility, but such a prosecution is not totally unforeseeable. In November 1992, a press report appeared concerning a 51-year-old journalist who woke up in hospital after a 'deep scrape' operation to find that during the operation her womb and ovaries had been removed (*Sunday Times*, Nov 1992). The surgeon found a swelling in her abdomen, though it was not life-threatening condition, and had gone on to cut out her ovaries. He said that 'I thought at her age it was the wiser thing to remove them.' The woman took her case to the Director of Public Prosecutions, who considered prosecution.

Failure to obtain consent to treatment may amount to the crime of battery, a common law offence. Some types of battery cannot be consented to, such as prize fighting or beatings for sexual gratification (*R* v. *Donovan* [1934] QB 638 and *R* v. *Brown* [1994] 1 AC 212). However, it appears to be the case that reasonable surgical interference does not constitute an inherently unlawful action and no crime will be committed as long as the patient has consented to the operation being undertaken (*AG Ref (No. 6 of 1980)* [1981] QB 715). There is the possibility that serious surgical procedures may also constitute an offence under section 18 of the Offences Against the Person Act 1861. This section makes it an offence to cause grievous bodily harm 'unlawfully and maliciously' to a person with the intention of causing grievous bodily harm. A court is unlikely to find that an operation to improve the patient's health has been undertaken unlawfully.

Finally, there is the chance that an operation might be held to be unlawful regardless of consent because it constituted the crime of maim. This is an ancient crime which makes it an offence to perform an operation or give an injury which has the effect of permanently disabling/weakening a man. Skegg (1984) suggests that such a prosecution is unlikely to be successful even if it were to be brought. Firstly, most medical treatment does not have the effect of permanently disabling a man and rendering him less useful for fighting. Secondly, even if an operation did have that effect it may still be lawful if undertaken for therapeutic purposes. In a recent consultation paper which examines the scope of criminal liability in relation to consent to treatment, the Law Commission (1996) has recommended reform of the law to recognise the legality of the performance of medical procedures such as surgical operations.

Civil law liability

Battery

While a criminal prosecution may be brought it is far more likely that failure to obtain consent will lead to the patient suing for damages in the civil courts. This may be on the basis that either the treatment amounted to a battery or that the nurse or doctor was negligent in providing the patient with inadequate information. A battery refers to any unlawful touching. Consent is a defence to battery. But what amounts to consent? In *Chatterson v. Gerson* ([1981] QB 432) Bristow J. said:

> 'In my judgment once the patient is informed in broad terms of the nature of the procedure which is intended and has given her consent then that consent is real and the cause of action on which to base the claim is negligence not trespass.'

It is sufficient that the patient understands the type of operation which is to be performed. The patient doesn't have to be informed of all the potential risks and implications of the clinical procedure.

Treating on the basis of temporary incompetence

Consent is not required if treatment is necessary in an emergency. The patient brought in bleeding and unconscious to Accident & Emergency can be treated without his or her consent. If it was claimed that treatment was unlawful then the nurse could claim the defence that the treatment was 'necessary'.

If, during an operation, it is found that a patient is suffering from, for example, a life threatening tumour then this tumour may be removed if it is necessary to save the patient's life, even though the medical team do not have the patient's express consent to removal. But, while it is lawful to undertake treatment without consent where necessary to do so, how far does this principle extend? Guidance can be taken from two notable decisions in Canada. In *Marshall* v. *Curry* ([1933] 3 DLR 260) the plaintiff sought damages for battery against a surgeon. During a hernia operation the surgeon had removed a testicle. He claimed that the removal was necessary because otherwise the patient's life would have been in danger. The court held that the surgeon was correct to go ahead and it would have been unreasonable to have delayed removal by waiting to obtain the patient's consent, then undertaking a second operation.

But 'reasonableness' is a question of degree, and dependant upon the urgency with which the operation should be undertaken. This was illustrated in the later case of *Murray* v. *McMurchy* ([1942] 2 DLR 442). A woman underwent a caesarean section. While operating, the doctor found that the woman's uterus was in such a state that it would have been exceedingly dangerous for her to undergo another pregnancy. He decided to sterilise her there and then and tied her fallopian tubes. On recovering from the operation and discovering what had happened, the woman brought an action for battery. The court upheld her claim. They were of the view that the doctor should have postponed the sterilisation operation until after the patient's consent had been obtained. In view of the uncertainty as to what constitutes necessary treatment, nurses should be exceedingly careful before proceeding with treatment in the absence of consent, save in an emergency situation where it is required to preserve the patient's life.

The patient who refuses treatment

A nurse may be faced by a patient who refuses to consent to medical treatment, such as Jehovah's Witnesses who refuse blood transfusions on religious grounds. If the nurse goes ahead and gives treatment against the patient's wishes this may well amount to a battery. Take, for example, the Canadian case of *Malette* v. *Schumann* ([1990] 67 DLR (4th) 321). The plaintiff was brought into hospital after a road accident. A nurse found a card in her pocket identifying her as a Jehovah's Witness and requesting that she never be given a blood transfusion. Despite this the doctor went ahead and administered the transfusion. On recovering her health the patient brought an action for battery and was awarded some $20 000 damages.

But while this is the general rule the English courts have indicated there may be situations in which treating a patient against his or her express wishes may be lawful. In *Re T* ([1992] 4 All ER 649) T, a woman 34 weeks pregnant was taken to hospital after she had been involved in a road accident. She developed pneumonia and her condition deteriorated. While in hospital she was visited by her mother. Although T was not a Jehovah's Witness, her mother was. There was some discussion between T and the medical team treating her as to whether she should be given a caesarean section. After some time alone with her mother T stated clearly that she did not want a blood transfusion. T then gave birth to a stillborn child. T's condition subsequently deteriorated. The hospital went to the court and asked for a declaration stating whether it would be lawful for T to be given a transfusion should it prove necessary. The court granted the declaration.

The Master of the Rolls, Sir John Donaldson stressed that a patient's refusal to consent should lead those treating the patient to ask was the patient capable of refusing consent to that treatment? He emphasised that refusals varied in the degree of seriousness and the scope of the refusal must be considered: did it apply to all situations?; was it based upon assumptions which had not been realised? He recommended that consent forms should be redesigned so that the consequences of refusal were brought forcibly to the patient's attention. This is a very controversial judgment. Were it to be followed, nurses and other members of the health care team would have to scrutinise very carefully any decision to refuse treatment. The other judges in this case did not go so far as Lord Donaldson, preferring to base their decision upon the fact that T had made her decision under pressure from her mother. Where there is doubt as to the patient's capacity to refuse treatment Lord Donaldson stressed that the health care team should seek a declaration from the court.

In a case decided not long after that of *Re T*, *Re S* ([1992] 4 All ER 671) a medical team was again able to override a patient's decision to refuse treatment. S was 6 days overdue giving birth. The team treating her believed that there was a very grave risk of a rupture to the uterus were the pregnancy to continue in the normal way. Essentially the life of both the woman and the fetus were at stake if the caesarean did not go ahead. S, a born-again Christian, refused the procedure on the basis that the operation was against her religious beliefs. The hospital sought a declaration from the court. Sir Stephen Brown granted the declaration, though in a short expedited judgment. It is possible, however, that cases such as *Re S* can be seen in many ways as exceptional in that the court was assessing the interests of the woman and fetus. There have been a number of subsequent cases in which the courts have been prepared to authorise enforced caesareans and these are considered further in the discussion on reproductive choice in Chapter 11.

What is clear is that neither *Re T* nor *Re S* allow nurses or other health care professionals to force a competent patient to receive treatment simply because they believe that the patient has made a totally irrational decision. If there is real doubt as to whether to proceed against the patient's wishes and the patient's life is in danger, advice should be sought from the court as to the legality of proceeding with treatment. This issue is discussed in the context of decisions relating to the end of life in Chapter 12.

Using compulsion in health care - public health powers

Generally speaking, in order for clinical procedures to be lawful a patient must give consent freely. However, in some situations compulsion may be sought. In the next chapter, the operation of the Mental Health Act 1983 is examined. In addition, there are a number of powers relating to compulsory care in the context of public health. If a patient is suffering from a notifiable disease, then the Public Health (Control of Disease) Act 1984 s.37 allows such a patient to be forcibly removed to hospital. The order must be made by a magistrate. The statute applies to those persons suffering from notifiable diseases such as cholera or typhoid. While HIV or AIDS are not notifiable conditions, special regulations have extended the power to make an order to persons who are HIV positive or who have AIDS (Public Health (Control of Infectious Diseases) Act 1984). There are also provisions under the National Assistance Act 1948 section 48, which allow the removal of persons who are aged, infirm, suffering from chronic disease, who are incapacitated, from their homes to hospital. Removal can only be undertaken after a magistrates order has been obtained. This order allows removal for a period of up to 3 months. There is also a special provision allowing a person to be removed in an emergency for a period of up to 3 weeks (National Assistance (Amendment) Act 1951 s1(1)). This may be undertaken on the recommendation of the community physician if supported by another practitioner.

Negligence

Once the patient has been told in general terms what is involved in medical procedures then there will no longer be liability in battery. But the patient may claim that while s/he has been given a general explanation s/he has not been told of the risks of the treatment and that this amounts to negligence. In establishing negligence for failure to inform, the legal principles are the same as in any other negligence claim (see Chapter 2). The plaintiff must show that s/he was owed a duty, that there was a breach of duty and that damage resulted from that breach.

In English law there is no doctrine of 'informed consent'; no requirement to inform the patient of all risks. This was made clear by the courts in the case of *Sidaway* v. *Bethlem Royal Hospital Governors* ([1985] 1 All ER 643). Mrs Sidaway underwent an operation after having suffered for some time from a recurring pain in her neck, right shoulder and arm. The operation was performed by a senior neurosurgeon at the Bethlem Royal Hospital. Even if carried out with all due care and skill there was a 1–2% risk of damage to nerve root and spinal column. While the risk of damage to the spinal column was less that to the nerve root, the consequences were more severe.

The plaintiff was left severely disabled after the operation. She claimed that she had not been given adequate warning as to the risks of the operation and she sought damages for negligence. During the proceedings it was found that, while the surgeon had told the patient of the risks of damage to the nerve root, he had not told her of the risks of damage to the spinal column. In doing this, he had conformed with what in 1974 would have been accepted as standard medical practice by a responsible and skilled body of neurosurgeons. The House of Lords rejected the claim that the surgeon had acted negligently. The majority held that the test which the courts should use in deciding whether the advice given was negligent was the same as that used in deciding whether medical treatment was negligent - the *Bolam* test. This test provides that a doctor:

> '...is not guilty of negligence if he has acted in accordance with a practice accepted as proper by a responsible body of medical men.'

That does not mean, however, that the court will always accept the word of the health care professional as to which risks should and which should not be disclosed. Only one member of the court in *Sidaway*, Lord Diplock, unreservedly accepted the *Bolam* test. Lord Bridge said that a judge could disagree with the evidence given to him:

> 'I am of the opinion that the judge might in certain circumstances come to the conclusion that disclosure of a particular risk was so obviously necessary to an informed choice on the part of the patient that no reasonably prudent medical man would fail to make it.'

Lord Templeman stressed that it was for the court to decide whether the doctor had acted negligently or not.

However, while the court has the ultimate power to overrule the view of the responsible body of professional practice as to what risks should be disclosed, it will only be in very rare situations that a court will be prepared to do so. In *Maynard* v. *West Midlands Health Authority* ([1984] 1 WLR 643), for example, the trial judge preferred one body of professional medical opinion to another and was held to have been wrong to do so. Even if the body of professional practice is very small in number, 4 or 5 out of 250 specialists for example, the court will still be prepared to accept its opinion (*De Freitas* v. *O'Brien* [1995] 6 Med LR 108).

There may be some situations in which it is thought that the patient would be unable to cope if told all the details of the prognosis. In *Sidaway*, Lord Scarman indicated that in such a situation information may be withheld on therapeutic grounds, the so-called 'therapeutic privilege'. This approach is reflected by the UKCC (1996) in the document *Guidelines for Professional Practice.*

> 'If patients or clients do not want to know the truth it should not be forced upon them. You must be sensitive to their needs and must make sure that your communication is effective. The patient or client must be given a choice in the matter. To deny them that choice is to deny their rights and so reduce dignity and independence.'

The requirement that the standard of disclosure should be that which would be recognised by a competent body of health care professionals can be contrasted with the approach taken in certain other countries that have recognised the doctrine of 'informed consent'. In the United States case of *Canterbury* v. *Spence* ([1972] 464 F 2d 772), the court declared that:

> 'respect for the patient's right of self-determination on particular therapy demands a standard set by law for the physician rather than one which physicians may or may not impose on themselves.'

Several states adopted a standard of disclosure based upon the information which a 'prudent patient' would expect to receive. Whether such a test would make a radical difference to the amount of information a patient receives is open to question. It is interesting to note that in the United States, some courts have used the notion of therapeutic privilege to restrict the requirement to disclose. A broader duty of disclosure has also been recognised in the Australian case of *Rogers* v. *Whittaker* ([1993] 4 Med LR 79).

In only one recent case concerning information disclosure have the courts shown that they are prepared to depart from an accepted body of clinical opinion. In *Smith* v. *Tunbridge Wells* ([1994] 5 Med LR 334) the plaintiff, a young man, claimed that a surgeon had failed to warn him of the risk of impotence and bladder dysfunction in an operation he underwent to treat rectal prolapse in 1988. The rectal prolapse was a condition which, while it did not endanger the patient's life, was embarrassing and caused discomfort. The plaintiff claimed that he would have rejected the operation had he known of the risks of the procedure. The court held that even though in 1988 a body of surgeons may not have warned of the condition, failure to inform might still constitute negligence. While evidence was given to the effect that certain leading textbooks of the day did not refer to the risks, nevertheless data from similar operations existed from which the surgeon could have been expected to extrapolate. This in effect imposes quite a stringent duty. It remains unclear whether this approach will be followed in later cases.

The duty of disclosure required under the *Sidaway* test is not fixed. As the expectations of patients change as to their involvement in their treatment, so the levels of disclosure required of practitioners are likely to change. Furthermore, the information required to be provided may be affected by external factors. For instance, a directive from Europe now requires that explanation leaflets be enclosed in certain drug products and this may affect the duty of disclosure in the future (Dir. 92/27/EEC(L113/8)). In addition, the Clinical Negligence Scheme for Trusts requires in Risk Management Standard No. 7 (NST 1996) that:

> 'Appropriate information be provided to patients on the risks and benefits of the proposed treatment or investigation and the alternatives available, before a signature on a consent form is sought.'

They state a number of factors in relation to the obtaining of consent, including that:

'• There is a patient information available showing the risks/benefits of 20 common elective treatments.
- There is a policy/guideline stating that consent for elective procedures is to be obtained by a person capable of performing the procedure.
- There is a clear mechanism for patients to obtain additional information about their condition.'

These standards are likely to inform professional practice in the future.

The questioning patient

If a patient, on being told about the treatment which is to be undertaken, asks questions as to the risks of the treatment and any complications which may arise, to what extent is the nurse obliged to give a full answer? In *Sidaway*, it was suggested that there might be a duty to respond fully if the patient asked specific questions. For example, Lord Bridge said that:

> 'when questioned specifically by a patient of apparently sound mind about the risks involved in a particular procedure proposed, the doctor's duty must, in my opinion, be to answer both truthfully and as fully as the questioner requires.'

However, the statements made were only judicial opinions which did not relate to the decision in that case and so were *obitur* not binding.

In the later case of *Blyth* v. *Bloomsbury AHA* ([1987] (1993) 4 Med LR 151 CA) the court indicated that the *Bolam* test should also apply to this situation. The plaintiff, Mrs Blyth, was a qualified nurse. She went into hospital to give birth. After the birth she was given a vaccination against rubella and an injection of the contraceptive Depo-Provera. Mrs Blyth said that she did not want to be given Depo-Provera until she had been told about the side effects. At the trial her claims as to what information she had been given were disputed. Expert evidence put forward at the trial indicated that at that time it was the practice to inform the patient that Depo-Provera led to irregular bleeding but not to inform about the other side effects. Kerr L.J. said that there was no obligation to disclose all information when a question was asked; it was sufficient if the information given was that which would be given by a responsible body of clinical practitioners (the *Bolam* test). In responding to questions he stressed that the answer given should depend upon the circumstances, the nature of the information, its reliability and relevance, the condition of the patient, etc. In deciding what information should be given initially, the nurse would need to examine the patient to see if s/he is capable of comprehending the information. Nevertheless, the questioning patient must be treated with respect and his or her questions must be given a serious response.

While the general obligation regarding disclosure of information relates to the standard of the responsible body of clinical practice, should that standard apply to all types of medical procedure? This question came before the courts in the case of *Gold* v. *Haringey Health Authority* ([1987] 2 All ER 888). Mrs Gold underwent a sterilisation operation. The operation was unsuccessful. She brought an action claiming that the surgeon was negligent because she was not told of the risk that the sterilisation operation might be reversed naturally, nor the fact that a vasectomy operation upon her husband would have carried less risk of reversal. At the time she underwent her operation there was a body of medical opinion which supported giving further information, but also a body of medical opinion which supported what her surgeon had done.

At first instance, Schiemmann J. drew a distinction between the level of information which had to be given in cases involving therapeutic as opposed to non-therapeutic treatment. He said that a sterilisation operation was non-therapeutic treatment and as such the approach taken in *Sidaway* was not applicable. It was for the court to decide whether or not the person giving advice should mention the chance that the operation would not achieve the desired result. However, on appeal, this approach was rejected. In the Court of Appeal, Lloyd L.J. said that the *Bolam* test applied. He saw problems in trying to draw a line between advice given in relation to therapeutic treatment and non-therapeutic treatment. For example, a plastic surgeon carrying out a skin graft may be acting therapeutically, but he might not be if he were carrying out a facelift or some other cosmetic operation.

Causation

As with any negligence claim, if the patient can show that s/he was given inadequate information by the nurse treating her or him, the patient must still go on to show that the failure to provide such information as to the risks of a particular clinical procedures *caused* the harm that s/he suffered. The court will ask, 'If this patient here had been given the information which she should have been given then would she have decided to go ahead with the treatment?'(*Chatterson* v. *Gerson* [1981] QB 432).

Providing information: professional conflicts over disclosure

In some situations the nurse may be of the view that a doctor or another nurse treating the patient has not provided the patient with adequate information or that the patient has not understood the information given. What should the nurse do? In the document *Guidelines for Professional Practice*, the UKCC (1996ii) states that:

> 'Sometimes you may not be responsible for obtaining the patient's or client's consent as, although you are caring for the patient or client you would not actually be carrying out the procedure. However, you are often best placed to know about the emotions, concerns and views of the patient or client and may be best able to judge what information is needed so that it is understood. With this in mind you should tell the other members of the health care team if you are concerned about the patient's or client's understanding of the procedure or treatment, for example, due to language difficulties.'

What if the nurse draws the doctor's/other nurse's attention to the perceived problem but they disagree with her? What should she do? The UKCC (1996iii) states that:

> 'There is potential for disagreement or even conflict between different professionals and relatives over giving information to a patient or client. When discussing these matters with colleagues or relatives, you must stress that your personal accountability is firstly to the patient and client. Any patient or client can feel relatively powerless when they do not have full knowledge about their care or treatment. Giving patients and clients information helps to empower them. For this reason, the importance of telling the truth cannot be over-estimated.'

The standard of disclosure laid down by the courts is that of the responsible body of professional clinical practice. If, for example, a doctor had given a patient the amount of information which a body of professional opinion would believe was sufficient, then he would have acted lawfully even though the nurse may disagree with the amount of information which has been given. It is very unlikely that the court would go against the approach which the doctor has taken.

Should the nurse inform the patient her- or himself? If s/he does then she may be put at risk of being disciplined for overstepping authority and disobeying the doctor. It is also possible that the doctor may be withholding the information for a specific reason, such as on therapeutic grounds, and the patient may not be able to cope with the information once given and may actually suffer harm. In such a situation, the nurse is at risk of an action subsequently being brought against her or him in negligence. The court would examine the nurse's actions and determine whether her or his conduct was such as would be supported by a responsible body of professional nursing practice.

If the nurse fails to act and the patient suffers harm then the nurse may also be at risk of legal proceedings. However, were proceedings to be brought against the nurse, s/he could claim to be simply following the doctor's orders. In earlier cases the courts have been willing to find that a nurse was not negligent because s/he had been following the orders of the doctor (*Gold* v. *Essex CC* [1942] 2 All ER 237). However, with the increasing autonomy of the nurse and the growth of professional practice, whether this approach would be given unreserved acceptance may be questioned.

In practice, should this situation arise it is suggested that the nurse should not go ahead and disclose immediately. S/he should ask the doctor why more information is not being given. If the doctor gives what the nurse regards to be an inadequate reason, then the matter should be referred to her or his line manager.

Concluding comments

The principles of consent to treatment outlined in this chapter underpin much of health care law. Matters of consent are considered in the chapters on reproductive choice, medical research and end of life. In the following chapter, consent in relation to two particular groups of patient, child patients and the mentally ill, are considered.

References

BMA/Law Society (1996) *Assessment of Mental Capacity: Guidance for Doctors and Lawyers: A report of the British Medical Association and the Law Society.* British Medical Association, London.

Brazier, M. (1991) 'Competence, consent and proxy consents.' In *Protecting the Vulnerable* (eds M. Brazier and M. Lobjoit). Routledge, London.

Clinical Negligence Scheme for Trusts (1996) *Risk Management Standards and Procedures, Manual of Guidance* CNST, Bristol.

Department of Health (1992) *Patient Consent to Examination or Treatment.* Appendix A(1). National Health Service Management Executive, HSG 92(32). DOH, London.

Grubb, A. (1994) 'Treatment without consent: adult' *Medical Law Review*, **2**, 92.

Kennedy, I. (1991) 'Consent to treatment.' In *Doctors, Patients and the Law* (ed. C. Dyer). Blackwell Scientific, Oxford.

Kennedy, I. and Grubb, A. (1994) *Medical Law: Text and Materials*, 2nd edn. Butterworths, London.

Law Commission (1996) *Consent in the Criminal Law: A Consultation Paper.* No. 139. HMSO, London.

Law Commission (1995) *Mental Incapacity.* Law Comm Report No. 231. HMSO, London, (i) para 3.2; (ii) para 3.12; (iii) para 3.16; (iv) para 3.18; (v) para 3.28; (vi) para 4.37.

Lord Chancellor's Department (1996) Press release 16 January and *Family Law* (1995) 246.

Skegg, P.D.G. (1984) *Law Medicine and Ethics.* Oxford University Press, Oxford.

UKCC (1996) *Guidelines for Professional Practice.* United Kingdom Central Council for Nursing, Midwifery and Health Visiting, London. (i) para 29.

UKCC (1993) *AIDS and HIV Infection: a UKCC Statement.* (Registrar's letter 6 April). United Kingdom Central Council for Nursing, Midwifery and Health Visiting, London, (i) para 25; (ii) para 29.

Chapter 6

Consent to treatment II: Children and the mentally ill

Jean McHale

In the previous chapter the basic principles of the law as it relates to consent to treatment were examined. This chapter focuses on the treatment of two particular groups of patients, children and the mentally ill. The basis on which treatment may be given and from whom consent to treatment should be obtained is examined in relation to the child patient. Particular difficult treatment issues arise with the child patient, as with the adult counterpart, in the context of treatment refusal. These issues are further complicated in the context of the child patient where conflicts arise between child and parent. The second part of the chapter considers legal regulation of treatment of the mentally ill patient in hospital and the community. Here, a statutory regime exists which regulates treatment procedures in the form of the Mental Health Act 1983.

Treating the child patient

Where the nurse is treating a child patient s/he must take care to ensure that the appropriate consent has been obtained. Where a child is very young, consent must be obtained from the person with 'parental responsibility'. This may be the child's mother, married father and unmarried father (s2 and s4 Children Act 1989) (with agreement with the mother or where a court order has been made giving him that power), a person holding a residence order (s12), or a local authority (s33). But there may be situations in which there is not sufficient time to consult a person with parental responsibility. For example, a child on her way to school is injured by a hit and run driver. She is taken to hospital bleeding profusely, in a critical condition. In an emergency, such treatment may be given as is immediately necessary, without parental consent being obtained. In addition, a child minder or a teacher has the right to do what is 'reasonable in all the circumstances' of the case for the purpose of safeguarding or promoting the child's welfare. This would include authorising medical treatment (s3(5) Children Act 1989). The Family Law Reform Act 1969 gives children who are 16 years and over the right to give consent themselves to surgical, medical or dental treatment (s8 Family Law Reform Act 1969).

Many uncertainties remain, however, as to what exactly constitutes 'treatment' for these purposes. It is obvious that the plaster on the wound, the surgery on the car accident victim are covered. What is less clear is the extent to which procedures ancillary to treatment are lawful. A difficult issue concerns the use of constraints upon young children, e.g. holding down a child to give treatment. It is submitted that wherever possible treatment should be given with the cooperation of the child and that the use of compulsion should be contemplated only in highly exceptional circumstances. Generally the performance of non-therapeutic procedures on a child create difficulties because often they cannot be said to be in the child's best interests. One approach is to say that certain procedures are justifiable as long as they are not against the child's best interests (*S* v. *McC*, *W* v. *W* [1972] AC24). Whether parents can consent to involvement in certain non-therapeutic procedures such as organ donation or involvement in clinical research are discussed further in later chapters.

The parental power of consent does not cover whatever treatment they believe to be in the child's best interests. Any treatment given is ultimately dependent upon the health professional's assessment of whether that treatment is appropriate for the child. Secondly, certain procedures are unlawful *per se*. For example, a mother cannot consent to her daughter being circumcised, because this practice was made illegal by the Prohibition of Female Circumcision Act 1985.

When is the child competent to consent to medical treatment?

As seen above, there is a statutory right for children aged 16 years and over to consent to medical or dental treatment. However, some children reach maturity earlier than others - 16 years is an arbitrary point. A young girl approaches a school nurse and wants advice because she intends obtaining the contraceptive pill. What is the legal position? Can such a girl be given such medication without parental consent? In *Gillick* v. *West Norfolk and Wisbech AHA* ([1985] 3 All ER 402), the House of Lords clearly stated that even if a child was under 16 years of age s/he may be able to give consent to medical treatment. In this case Mrs Victoria Gillick sought a declaration that the DHSS had been wrong to issue a direction indicating that a doctor might give contraceptive advice/treatment to a child under 16 years without parental consent. The House of Lords, by a narrow majority, dismissed her claim. Lord Fraser held that a doctor would be justified in giving a girl contraceptive advice without her parent's knowledge and/or consent. He suggested a number of factors to be taken into account in making such an assessment. These included that: the doctor is satisfied that the girl would understand his advice; he has been unable to persuade her to tell her parents or to let him tell her parents; the girl is likely to begin having intercourse with/without contraceptive treatment; without contraceptive advice/treatment her physical or mental health could suffer and that it would be in the girl's best interests to receive contraceptive assistance without her parent's consent.

Another member of the House of Lords, Lord Scarman, saw the issue in terms of the rights of the child:

> 'as a matter of law the parental right to determine whether or not a minor child below the age of 16 will have medical treatment terminates if and when the child achieves a sufficient understanding and intelligence to enable him to understand fully what is proposed. It will be a question of fact whether a child seeking advice has sufficient understanding of what is involved to give a consent valid in law. (p. 423)'

Two members of the House of Lords, Lords Brandon and Templeman, dissented. Lord Templeman said that there are many things that a girl under 16 years needs to practice but sex is not one of them.

After the *Gillick* decision it is clear that a child under 16 years may consent to medical treatment if s/he is judged to be competent to give that consent. The difficulty with the test laid down in *Gillick* is that it means that a nurse treating a child patient has the task of assessing whether this particular child is competent to consent to *this particular* treatment. A child may have sufficient maturity to consent to one type of treatment, such as treatment for cuts and bruises, while at the same time not being competent to decide about another type of treatment, such as an operation. It must be emphasised that even if a child is under 16 years, good practice would dictate that, wherever possible, an effort should be made to involve the child in any decisions regarding care and treatment.

Court orders

The vast majority of treatment decisions are straightforward and will present no legal difficulties as long as the nurse complies with the general legal principles in relation to disclosure of information set out in the previous chapter, and if she obtains consent from the appropriate person. There are, however, some situations in which difficult dilemmas arise. The health care professionals may be uncertain as to what action to take. There are three main routes through which an application may be made to the court. The case may be referred under what is known as the court's 'inherent jurisdiction'; the court has a power to make orders regarding medical treatment. The child may be made a ward of court. This power was limited by the Children Act 1989 and today a local authority cannot apply for wardship, although other interested bodies such as a health authority may do so. In addition, wardship cannot be sought if the child is in local authority care. The third option is to ask the court to make one of two orders created by the Children Act 1989. The first of these is a 'prohibited steps' order; this has the effect of stopping a parent exercising his or her parental responsibility without the consent of the court. Secondly, an application could be made for a 'specific issue order'. This involves asking the court to give directions on a specific question before it, for example, giving consent to treatment (s8). In making an order the court considers whether the child's welfare dictates that the treatment be undertaken.

Refusal of treatment by those with parental responsibility

What if a course of treatment is proposed for a critically ill child but the parents refuse to give their consent? Can treatment be given? The parents may be refusing treatment for a particular reason, such as their own ethical or religious beliefs. In such circumstances health care professionals should hesitate before treating. The impact upon the child, were treatment to be authorised in the face of parental opposition, requires some consideration. Were treatment to be given in such a situation, this may have the effect that the child is alienated from his or her own family. The action taken is likely to relate to the urgency with which treatment is required. If a child is literally bleeding to death then, it is suggested, it is justifiable to treat, even in the face of parental opposition.

But if, while a child's life is in grave danger, death is not imminent, then the matter may be referred to the court by the hospital or by the local authority under the court's inherent jurisdiction, or through a specific issue order asking for clarification of their legal position in undertaking treatment.

Such an issue came before the courts in the case of *Re S (a minor)* ([1993] 1 FLR 376). A four and a half year old child was suffering from T-cell leukaemia with a high risk that death would occur. Chemotherapy was offered but this required a blood transfusion. S's parents, who were dedicated Jehovah's Witnesses, refused to consent to the treatment. The local authority went to court and asked for an order under its inherent jurisdiction and the parents asked for a prohibited steps order. In authorising treatment Thorpe J. noted that the parents' refusal of treatment would deny their son the 50% chance of survival which was offered by the therapy. It had been suggested that one reason why treatment should not be given was that the child would have to live for years to come with parents who 'believed that his life was prolonged through an ungodly act'. Thorpe J. recognised that by providing the child with a transfusion there was a further risk of conflict between child and parent. However, as the judge said:

> 'The reality seems to me that family reactions will recognise that the responsibility of consent was taken from them, and as a judicial act, absolved their conscience of responsibility.'

In the case of *Re O (a minor) (Medical Treatment)* ([1993] 2 FLR 149), a baby was born prematurely. The child suffered from a respiratory distress syndrome, which meant that she would require a blood transfusion. The parents were Jehovah's Witnesses and were opposed to the transfusion. Other options were tried but it was realised that a blood transfusion was inevitable. The inherent jurisdiction of the High Court was invoked. Johnson J. gave directions to the effect that if medical advice deemed it necessary the child should be given a blood transfusion.

A more recent and contrasting case provides an illustration of judicial willingness to support a parent's decision to refuse treatment. In *Re T* ([1997] 1WLR 242), a child was born with a liver defect which was life threatening. An operation had initially been carried out on the child at the age of three and a half months which had been unsuccessful and had resulted in the child suffering a great deal of pain. The child then needed a liver transplant. At the time of the hearing both child and parents were in a foreign country. The parents, who were health care professionals, were opposed to the treatment being undertaken. The mother did not want the child to undergo the suffering that this procedure would involve. The operation was not available in the Commonwealth country where the treatment was being given, and had an order been made the parents would have had to bring the child back to this country for treatment.

At first instance, the judge held that leave should be given to the health professionals to perform the operation despite parental opposition. In the Court of Appeal this order was reversed. Butler Sloss L.J. examined a number of cases involving the decision to treat the incompetent minor. She noted the exceptional nature of this case and stated that:

> 'This mother and child are one for the purpose of this unusual case and the decision of the court to consent to the operation jointly affects the mother and son and it also affects the father. The welfare of this child depends upon his mother.'

The decision of the Court of Appeal in *Re T* has proved controversial. The court placed great weight on the views of the parents. This case may appear to run contrary to a number of cases concerning refusal of treatment by parents on religious grounds, where the views of the parents have been overridden by the courts. Emphasis was placed upon the fact that the parents were health professionals. Does this place the opinions of such parents in a special category apart from those of parents generally - even where the parents possess deep religious convictions? While the decision of the Court of Appeal in *Re T* has attracted considerable public attention it's wider implications remain to be assessed. In *Re T* the court emphasised the unusual nature of this case and the close emotional attachment which existed between the mother and baby. It may be speculated as to whether the location of the parties may have had some influence on the ultimate decision reached, as the parents were abroad at the time. There are a number of cases in which the court has granted orders allowing active treatment to be withheld from newly born infants and these cases are explored in Chapter 12 below.

When can treatment be given in the face of a child's refusal?

Parents bring their son to be vaccinated. The boy goes into the treatment room but then begins to scream and refuses to let the nurse touch him. Can he be compelled to have the injection? In the case of a very young child, while actually giving this injection may not be very easy, in strict law the parent may consent to treatment despite the child's refusal. However, in practice, the nurse may suggest to the parents that s/he does not go ahead at that time but that they bring the child back another day. Difficult issues arise in relation to older children who are assessed as *Gillick* competent. Such a child may be able to *consent* to medical treatment but what if s/he refuses? Can treatment be given and if so on what basis? In the professional role as patient advocate the nurse is required to respect the autonomy of her patient, which includes providing support for a patient who decides to refuse treatment or that treatment should be withdrawn (UKCC, 1996i). Nonetheless it has been noted that in law the power of the adult patient to refuse treatment is not unlimited (see Chapter 5). As far as the child patient is concerned it is clearly the case that the right to refuse treatment is again not absolute. It is also likely that where a child *refuses* treatment this will mean that, as with the adult patient, a more rigorous assessment is made of that child's competence.

The Court of Appeal has indicated that if a competent child refuses treatment, his or her parents may override this refusal. In *Re R* ([1991] 4 All ER 177 CA) Lord Donaldson said that the fact that a child was competent to consent to treatment did not mean that all parental rights were removed. Once a child reaches maturity s/he receives a key to the door of treatment. However, the child's parents have keys and they keep the key once the child gains maturity. A parent can authorise treatment even though the child refuses. Lord Donaldson's words in that case were *obiter* and the other members of the Court of Appeal did not agree with his approach.

However, in the later case of *Re W* ([1992] 3 WLR 758) the Court of Appeal confirmed that the parents could lawfully override the refusal of a competent child. This case concerned an anorexic 16-year-old girl who opposed removal to a treatment centre where it was likely that an active treatment regime might be imposed. The court held that although she was competent to consent to treatment, her refusal could be overridden. Lord Donaldson moved away from the keyholder analogy and instead said that a doctor acquires a legal 'flak jacket' as protection from being sued when he receives consent from a child over 16, a *Gillick* competent child or from a person with parental responsibility. He went on to say:

> 'No minor of whatever age has power by refusing consent to treatment to override a consent to treatment by someone who has parental responsibility for the minor. Nevertheless such a refusal was a very important consideration in making clinical judgements and for parents and the court in deciding themselves whether to give consent.'

The judgment in this case was contrary to general opinion as to the interpretation of the *Gillick* case and the Family Law Reform Act 1969. However, at present, even if a *Gillick* competent child refuses medical treatment it appears that his or her parents may override the refusal. However, the court in *Re W* suggested that before a major surgical procedure is undertaken on a child against her will it is desirable for the issue to be referred to the court. The court would then determine what is in the child's best interests, taking into account the child's expressed wishes and the strength of the child's beliefs. It may be, for example, that while a child has strong convictions at present, this may be only a passing phase. The urgency of the treatment is also a relevant factor.

In *Re W* Nolan L.J. suggested that the court could intervene where the child's welfare was 'threatened by serious and imminent risk that the child will suffer grave and irreversible mental or physical harm', while Balcombe L.J. stated that the court should only intervene where refusal would lead to the child's death.

Children were given certain statutory rights to refuse court ordered assessment and treatment under the Children Act 1989. This may seem rather at odds with the approach of the courts in *Re R* and *Re W*. However, in the case of *South Glamorgan CC* v. *W and B* ([1993] 1 FLR 574) the court confirmed that a court still possessed certain residual powers under its inherent jurisdiction to override a child's refusal. The decision in this case has been criticised on the basis that it goes against clear words of statute.

Authorisation of treatment in the face of a child's opposition may also give rise to problems as to the relationship between the powers to compulsorily treat under the Mental Health Act 1983 (which will be considered later) and the powers at common law. In *Re K, W and H (minors) (Medical Treatment)*([1993] FLR 584), advance parental consent was required before children were admitted for treatment in a specialist psychiatric institution. Three children were admitted. They later complained as to their treatment including the administration of emergency medication. An action was brought before the court under section 8 of the Children Act 1989 to clarify the legality of the treatment of these three children. Two were 15 years old and were suffering from unsocialised adolescent conduct disorder; the other child, who was almost 15 years, was suffering from bi-polar affective disorder. Thorpe J. said that none of the children was *Gillick* competent but that even if they were, the doctor had received parental authorisation of treatment in the form of the advance consents before they had entered the psychiatric institution, and thus was justified in law in going ahead and providing treatment. He commented that a specific issue order to authorise treatment under section 8 of the Children Act 1989 was not required where parental consent existed. The difficulty with such an approach is that it denies children the safeguards in the form of the statutory provisions limiting provision of treatment contained in the Mental Health Act 1983 (Bate, 1995).

While certain powers are given to courts and parents to override the decisions of competent children, these powers should be used only in exceptional circumstances. Generally it is not clinically beneficial to treat a child where s/he is objecting, particularly where this involves detention against a child's will.

Refusal of treatment by both children and parents

What if both parents and child patient are in agreement in their opposition to treatment and emphasise that this is on religious grounds? In such a situation the consequences of refusal of treatment should be clearly explained to the child. Dilemmas may arise, however, where that refusal is likely to result in the patient's death. It may be the case that the child's will is being overborne, but equally the child may have a fundamental religious belief and have reached his or her own decision to refuse treatment based on that belief. In such a situation where refusal of treatment would have the consequence that death would result, an application to the court would be appropriate, to ask for the authorisation of treatment.

This issue came before the courts in the case of *Re E (minor) (Wardship: Medical Treatment)* ([1993] 1 FLR 386). A was fifteen and three quarters years old and was suffering from leukaemia. A's parents were devout Jehovah's Witnesses, and both A and his parents were opposed to a blood transfusion. Consent was given to therapy, which avoided a blood transfusion, but which only had a 40–50% chance of full remission as opposed to 80-90% had treatment which involved a blood transfusion been given. The health authority made an application to the court when it became apparent that within a matter of hours blood platelet levels would fall to unacceptable levels and A was at risk of a stroke or heart attack. The judge, Ward J., stated that although A was a calm and intelligent person, in his view he did not really understand the implications of his decision.

> 'I am quite satisfied that A does not have any sufficient comprehension of the pain he has yet to suffer, of the fear that he will be undergoing, of the distress not only occasioned by that fear but also - and more importantly - the distress he will inevitably suffer as he, a loving son, helplessly watches his parents' and his family's distress. They are a close family and a brave family, but I find that he has no realisation of the full implications that lie before him as to the process of dying.'

While noting A's religious convictions he stated:

> 'I respect this boy's profession of faith but I cannot discount at least the possibility that he may in later years suffer some diminution in his convictions. There is no settled certainty about matters of this kind.'

This type of case poses difficult questions. While the views of the child may very well change, equally they may not. The minor in *Re E* died subsequently when on reaching the age of 18 years he refused treatment.

Seeking treatment and care when a child is being neglected or put at risk

A health visitor believes that a child is being neglected by his parents or that he is being abused. What can the health visitor do? Her or his actions will obviously depend upon the gravity of the situation and the child's need for immediate care. If a child is suffering from a particular medical condition and it is believed that the child still needs care, what can be done? In this situation the matter should be referred to Social Services. All local authorities and county councils have child protection policies which should be consulted by health care professionals. The local authority may decide to instigate an investigation. The health visitor would be consulted while any investigation was being undertaken. Measures may be taken to bring the child under the care or supervision of the local authority. These are matters which go beyond the scope of this book and readers are referred to specialist texts on the subject.

Treating the mentally ill patient

In Chapter 5 the question of treatment of mentally incompetent patients was examined. Here, the question of treatment of the mentally ill patient is considered. Mental illness and mental incompetence should not be equated. A mentally ill person may be perfectly competent to consent to involvement in some clinical procedures, for example involvement in clinical research, even though he or she has diminished competence in relation to other matters.

It is important for the nurse to be aware of the operation of the Mental Health Act 1983, not only if s/he intends to specialise in mental health nursing, but also because issues involving treatment of the mentally ill arise in a wide variety of nursing situations. The nurse should also be aware of the Mental Health Act Code of Practice. This is not legally binding but provides an indication of good practice. For fuller discussion of this area the nurse is referred to specialist texts dealing with mental health law (Dimond, 1996; Hogget 1996). We are focusing on treatment given after detention under civil law power. Powers of detention are also available in the context of the criminal law.

Admission into hospital for treatment

A mentally disordered patient may be informally admitted to a hospital for psychiatric treatment. Such a patient may refuse any treatment and may leave hospital freely at any time (s131 Mental Health Act 1983). Any attempt to detain the patient may lead to a civil law claim for damages for false imprisonment being brought. It appears that the use of 'constraints' such as special locks on doors to prevent patients wandering out on to the street is lawful (Hoggett, 1997). However, as Hoggett notes 'consideration should be given to "sectioning" people who persistently and purposefully try to leave' (p. 143).

The Mental Health Act Code of Practice (1993) indicates that, wherever possible, preference should be given to informal admission. But in some situations it is necessary to compulsorily admit a patient. Considered first below is the basis on which a patient can be brought from the community into hospital and given treatment and second, the grounds for detaining a patient who is presently in a hospital on an informal basis.

Emergency removal under the Mental Health Act 1983

The Mental Health Act 1983 contains emergency powers enabling a person to be removed to hospital for treatment. Section 135 of the Act provides that a magistrate may authorise a warrant allowing a police officer to gain entry to premises and remove a person to a 'place of safety'. The warrant will be granted if a magistrate is satisfied that the person is suffering from mental disorder and 'has been or is being ill-treated, neglected or kept otherwise than under proper control, or is living alone and is unable to care for themselves'. When entering premises the Act requires a police officer to be accompanied by an approved social worker and a doctor. A person may only be detained under Section 135 for up to 72 hours. After this point any continued detention must be authorised under one of the other powers contained in the Mental Health Act 1983.

Power of police to remove a person found in a public place

A man is found wandering in the street showing clear signs of mental disorder. If a policeman believes that the man is in immediate need of care/control, he may remove him to a 'place of safety', such as a hospital, for up to 72 hours (s136 Mental Health Act 1983). The powers under Section 136 apply to 'any place to which the public has access'. They enable an individual to be examined by a doctor and interviewed by an approved social worker as a preliminary to providing care or admission to hospital for treatment under the Mental Health Act 1983. The operation of this section has come under considerable criticism, with claims that the section has been inadequately supervised and details of patients admitted under the section being inadequately recorded.

At present, if a person opposes removal from his or her home and treatment is needed, there is no alternative but forcible removal to hospital under the Mental Health Act 1983. The Law Commission has proposed a new power to allow the removal of a vulnerable person 'at risk' from his or her home (Law Commission, 1995i). This would be for the purpose of an assessment order or a temporary protection order being made, enabling removal to protective accommodation for a period of up to 10 days.

Admission for assessment

Section 2 of the Mental Health Act 1983 allows a patient to be admitted for 'assessment'. Section 2 applies to patients suffering from a mental disorder justifying detention in hospital at least for a limited period. It must also be shown that detention is needed in the interests of the patient's own health and safety or to protect others. The application must be made by the patient's 'nearest relative' or by an approved social worker. The approved social worker should inform the nearest relative that an application is being made (s11(3)). The application must be supported by two doctors, one of whom must have been approved by the Secretary of State as having special experience in the treatment of mental disorder. The 'nearest relative' is defined in the Act as being the relative who usually lives with that patient or the person with the closest connection as determined in relation to a long list of relatives - in order of priority. The approved social worker is a social worker appointed to work under the Mental Health Act. Section 2 is intended to provide a short term detention with the limited purpose of determining suitability for continued assessment (*R* v. *Wilson and Williamson* [1995] *The Independent*, 19 April). Admission under this section is for a period of up to 28 days. This is a one-off admission, as the period cannot be renewed.

'Mental disorder' under this section is defined as 'mental illness, arrested or incomplete development of mind, psychopathic disorder and any other disability of mind s1(2). The Act does not define mental illness but the courts have indicated that it should be given its ordinary meaning (*W* v. *L* [1974] QB 711). This is commonly known as 'the man must be mad' test (Hoggett, 1996). The definition of mental disorder expressly excludes sexual deviations and alcoholism (s1(3) Mental Health Act 1983). Psychopathic disorder refers to a disorder/disability of mind (whether or not including significant impairment of intelligence) resulting in abnormally aggressive or seriously irresponsible conduct.

Admission for treatment

A person may be admitted for treatment for longer periods under section 3 of the Mental Health Act 1983. Application for admission under this section may be made by the same persons as under section 2. It must be shown that the patient is suffering from 'mental illness, severe mental impairment, psychopathic disorder or mental impairment' (s 3(2)). Mental impairment refers to arrested/incomplete mental development including significant impairment of intelligence/social functioning and associated with abnormally aggressive/seriously irresponsible conduct. The condition must be of a nature such that it is appropriate for the patient to receive treatment in a hospital.

Where treatment is sought for psychopathic disorder or mental impairment it must be shown that the treatment is likely to alleviate or prevent deterioration in the patient's condition, though it is not necessary to show that it would provide a guaranteed cure. Treatment may include nursing and rehabilitation including group therapy which could result in the patient being rendered more cooperative (*R* v. *Canons Park Mental Health Review Tribunal Ex parte A* ([1994] 1 All ER 481). Finally, it must be shown that admission is necessary for the patient's health and safety or for the protection of other persons and that necessary treatment cannot be given unless the patient is detained under this section. Admission under Section 3 allows the patient to be detained for up to 6 months. This period can be renewed, initially for 6 months, then on an annual basis.

Emergency power - section 4

In an emergency a patient can be admitted under section 4 of the Mental Health Act 1983 if one doctor certifies that s/he is suffering from 'mental disorder'. The doctor should, if possible, already know the patient. A doctor who certifies admission under section 4 does not have to be a specialist in mental illness. The person making the application should have examined the patient in the previous 24 hours. Section 4 allows detention for up to a maximum of 72 hours. This period can be extended by conversion into 'admission for assessment' under section 2 .

Detaining a patient in hospital

In some situations it becomes obvious that a patient receiving care in hospital on a voluntary basis requires compulsory detention. The Mental Health Act 1983 contains powers to allow a patient to be detained to enable assessment of whether prolonged detention is necessary. One of these powers applies expressly to the nurse. Section 5(4) of the Mental Health Act 1983 gives the nurse power to detain an in-patient, if the nurse is of the view that the patient is suffering from a mental disorder to such a degree that it is necessary for the patient to be immediately restrained from leaving hospital, and a doctor is unable to examine the patient at that time.

The power applies to nurses on part 3 or part 5 or parts 13 or 14 of the statutory Register (part 3 includes first level nurses trained in nursing people suffering from mental illness; part 5 first level nurses trained in nursing those suffering from mental handicap; part 13 nurses who have obtained qualifications after following a course of mental health nursing; and part 14 those qualified from a course of mental handicap nursing). If the nurse decides to exercise this power s/he must record this fact in writing. Detention under section 5(4) is limited to 6 hours or to the point at which the doctor can see the patient. This is an important power - and one the nurse should use with discretion. There is a danger that, as Unsworth notes, the nurse may be seen as 'gaoler' rather than carer (Unsworth, 1987).

The Mental Health Act Code of Practice sets out a number of criteria which a nurse should take into account before exercising power under section 5(4) (para 9.2). The nurse should consider:

'1. The likely arrival time of the doctor as against the likely intention of the patient to leave. Most patients who express a wish to leave hospital can be persuaded to wait until a doctor arrives to discuss it further. Where this is not possible, the nurse must try to predict the impact of any delay upon the patient.
2. The consequences of a patient leaving hospital immediately - the harm that might occur to the patient or others - taking into account:
   (a) What the patient says he will do
   (b) Likelihood of the patient committing suicide
   (c) Patient's current behaviour and in particular any changes in usual behaviour
   (d) Likelihood of the patient behaving in a violent manner
   (e) Any recently received messages from relatives or friends
   (f) Any recent disturbance on the ward (which may or may not involve the patient)
   (g) Any relevant involvement of other patients.
3. The patient's known unpredictability and any other relevant information from other members of the multidisciplinary team.'

The wording of section 5(4) appears to assume that a nurse should complete the forms before detaining the patient. But does this mean that the patient cannot be detained until the forms have been completed? The question is not expressly dealt with in the 1983 Act. At common law there were powers allowing the insane to be arrested. It is uncertain how far these powers still exist though; in one view sufficient common law powers do exist justifying such detention (*Black v. Forsey* (1988) *The Times*, 21 May).

The section requires that detention must be authorised by suitably qualified nurses - RMN or a RNMH. But what if there are no suitably qualified nurses on the ward? The Code of Practice provides that if it is likely that section 5(4) might be used, then:

> 'they should ensure that suitable arrangements are in place for a suitably qualified nurse to be available should the power need to be invoked.'

Nevertheless there is still the possibility that a nurse brought in to exercise the power may not have a sufficiently thorough knowledge of that particular patient (Gunn, 1994). The holding power under Section 5(4) applies for a maximum of 6 hours.

Detention may be authorised under Section 5(2) by a doctor. The doctor must provide the hospital managers with a report as to why s/he believes that the patient's detention is required. Once the managers have obtained a copy of the report then detention can be authorised for a period of up to 72 hours. It should be noted that this power applies to *in-patients* as opposed to patients simply visiting the hospital for treatment. It should be noted that while Section 5(2) powers can be applied to any in-patient as long as the relevant criteria are satisfied, Section 5(4) can be used by a nurse only in relation to a patient receiving treatment for a mental disorder as an inpatient.

It should be emphasised that sections 5(4) and 5(2) are holding powers to allow detention and assessment prior to possible authorisation of longer detention under one of the other provisions of the 1983 Act.

Providing the patient with information

A detained patient must be given information enabling him or her to understand the grounds for and conditions for detention (s132 Mental Health Act 1983). This duty is one which is likely to be delegated to the nurse. The patient must be informed of what provisions of the Mental Health Act 1983 s/he is being detained under, the right to apply to a mental health tribunal for discharge and how certain provisions of the Mental Health Act 1983, such as those relating to consent to treatment, affect him/her (s132 Mental Health Act 1983). This information must be given as soon as it is reasonably practicable to do so after detention has begun. Good practice dictates that the information should be given orally and in writing. There should be a procedure in existence stating who should give the patient the information.

Treatment of the detained patient

The Mental Health Act 1983 only regulates treatment given for the patient's mental disorder (s63), a mentally disordered person may still have capacity to give consent or refusal to other types of treatment. 'Treatment' includes medication and nursing care but may also extend to, for instance, feeding, if the patient's mental illness leads to the refusal of food (*B* v. *Croyden HA* [1995] 1 All ER 683). It has been suggested that the definition of mental illness includes anorexia nervosa. (Mental Health Act Commission Fourth Biennial Report and *Riverside Mental Health Trust* v. *Fox* [1994] 2 Med Law Review 95). In the case of a pregnant schizophrenic patient the court has also been prepared to hold that treatment may include the induction of labour and a caesarean section *(Tameside and Glossop Acute Services Trust* v. *CH*) *(a Patient)* ([1996] 1 FCR 753). It should be noted that even where a patient may be compelled to receive medication within 3 months under section 63, every attempt must be made to obtain the consent of the patient.

Psychosurgery/surgical implantation of hormones

Section 57 sets out a special procedure for psychosurgery and for other procedures governed by regulations including the surgical implantation of hormones. The patient must consent to the administration of this treatment.

In addition a second opinion approved doctor appointed by the Secretary of State and two other persons appointed by the Mental Health Act Commission must have:

> 'certified in writing that the patient is capable of understanding the nature, purpose and likely effects of the treatment in question and has consented to it. (s57(2)(a)).'

One of these persons must be a nurse and the other should be neither a nurse or doctor.

The second opinion approved doctor is appointed for these purposes by the body which regulates the conduct of the Mental Health Act, the Mental Health Commission. The doctor must also certify that 'having regard to the likelihood of the treatment alleviating or preventing a deterioration of the patient's condition the treatment should be given' (s57(2)(b)). These safeguards apply both to patients detained under the Mental Health Act 1983 and to informal patients.

Electroconvulsive therapy and administration of medicines after 3 months

The administration of medicines and electroconvulsive therapy (ECT) is governed by Section 58 of the 1983 Act. ECT may be appropriate, for instance, if a patient suffers from severe depression. As far as the administration of medicines is concerned, once 3 months have passed from the point when the patient was first admitted and given treatment for his or her mental disorder before the nurse may continue to administer any medicines requires special authorisation. The Code of Practice states that the

> 'period starts on the occasion when medication for mental disorder was first administered by any means during any period of continuous detention. The medication does not necessarily have to be administered continuously throughout the three month period. (para 16.11)'

Before ECT is given or medicines are administered after 3 months, one of two additional criteria must be satisfied. Either the patient must consent, with this consent being verified by the practitioner treating the patient or, if the patient refuses consent, treatment may still be given if authorised by a second opinion approved doctor.

The doctor must state that either the patient is not competent because he or she cannot understand the nature, purpose or likely effects of treatment or that, although the patient is competent and is refusing treatment, in view of the likelihood of it alleviating or preventing a deterioration in the patient's condition treatment should be given (s58(3)(b)). In forming his or her opinion, the second opinion approved doctor should also consult two other persons professionally involved in that person's care. The statute requires that at least one of these persons is a nurse (s58(4)). The grade of nurse is not specified. Again, the other person must be neither nurse nor doctor (s58(4)).

Treatment under sections 57 and 58 should be the subject of regular review. It should be noted that consents here are not always required on each separate occasion, it is sufficient that the consents relate to the overall plan of care (s59).

Treating in an emergency

In an emergency the safeguards contained in section 57 and section 58 may be bypassed under section 62 of the Act. Treatment may be given firstly if it is immediately necessary to save the patient's life. Secondly, treatment, which is not irreversible, may be given to alleviate serious suffering by the patient. Thirdly, treatment which is immediately necessary and represents the minimum interference necessary to prevent the patient from behaving violently or being a danger to him- or herself or others may be given if it is not irreversible or hazardous in nature. 'Irreversible' is defined as treatment entailing unfavourable physical or psychological consequences. 'Hazardous' refers to treatment which entails significant physical hazard. Gunn (1994) has suggested that those situations in which treatment may be given lawfully under this section are likely to be exceedingly limited. It is difficult to see how the performance of psychosurgery or surgical implantation of hormones can be justified in an emergency. Medication can, in any case, be given in the absence of the patient's consent within 3 months of a person first receiving medication for mental disorder during any continuous period of detention within 3 months of a person being sectioned. The only situation in which Gunn (1994) envisages use of section 62 is in an emergency to give ECT to a patient who is in a catatonic stupor and who might otherwise die.

It has been claimed that in some instances treatment given under section 62 has extended beyond what is justifiable within the provisions of the section. For example, there have been three reported cases in Broadmoor special hospital where patients have died following doses of antipsychotic medication in excess of the guide produced jointly by the BMA and the Royal Pharmaceutical Society of Great Britain (Fennell, 1994). A nurse who believes that the criteria laid down in the Mental Health Act 1983 are not being followed should make her or his concerns known to those who authorised this treatment. If necessary, the nurse should inform the line manager. Where an abuse has occurred, the line manager should inform the hospital authorities and make the Mental Health Act Commission aware of the situation.

Use of seclusion

The use of seclusion in mental hospitals came under scrutiny in the report into the abuses of mentally ill patients at Ashworth special hospital. Seclusion is defined in the Mental Health Code of Practice as:

> 'the supervised confinement of a patient alone in a room which may be locked for the protection of others from significant harm. (para 18.15)'

The Code of Practice emphasises that it must be used as a last resort.

The precise legality of seclusion is unclear. It may be lawful because it is the application of reasonable force which amounts to self-defence.

The Code of Practice provides that the nurse in charge of the ward may impose seclusion on a patient but where this is done a doctor should be immediately called (para 18.17). A number of criteria must be fulfilled. First, a nurse should be within sight and sound of the place where the patient is being held and should be present if the patient has been sedated (para 18.18). Second, the patient should be observed and a documented report should be made every 15 minutes as to whether seclusion is necessary (para 18.19). Third, if seclusion is continued then two nurses in the seclusion room should undertake a review every 2 hours and a doctor should review every 4 hours. Where the seclusion has continued for more than 8 hours consecutively or for more than 12 hours intermittently over 48 hours an independent review is required. This should be undertaken by a consultant 'or other doctor of suitable seniority' and a team of nurses and other health professionals, none of whom had been involved in the care of the patient when the original seclusion was undertaken (para 18.20).

Transfer

A patient detained under the Mental Health Act 1983 may be transferred to another unit managed by a different NHS trust or to a registered mental nursing home registered to take detained patients.

Discharging the patient

The period of detention may come to an end or the patient may leave as a result of being discharged. A trust or authority can discharge any patient who has been admitted for assessment or treatment at any time (s23). The decision to discharge is to be taken by a committee of three persons (s24(4)(5)). The nearest relative may also apply to the hospital for the patient's discharge (s23(2)(a)) and must give notice in writing (s25) . The patient has the right to apply for discharge to a mental health review tribunal (s66). In addition, an automatic reference will be made to a tribunal if the patient has not exercised the right to apply during the first 6 months of detention. Under section 68, automatic referral must be made if the patient has not been before the tribunal for 3 years. A Mental Health review tribunal (of which there are eight nationally) is a body comprised of three members, one legal, one medical and one lay. It is required to discharge patients if they are no longer suffering from mental disorder/illness or further detention is not required for the purposes of the patient's health or safety or to protect other persons. It may also exercise a discretion to discharge even if these criteria have not been satisfied.

Liability of the nurse under the Mental Health Act 1983

As long as a nurse acts in accordance with her or his statutory powers under the Mental Health Act 1983 then section 139 provides that:

> 'No person shall be liable...to any civil or criminal proceedings...in respect of any act purporting to be done in pursuance of this Act...unless the act was done in bad faith or without reasonable care.'

This limits the possibility of a civil action against the nurse (*Poutney* v. *Griffiths* [1975] 2 All ER 881). A patient may still bring an action challenging his or her detention under judicial review on the basis the health care professionals have acted outside their powers.

Treating mentally incapacitated persons in the community

Some patients suffering from a mental disorder may benefit from treatment in the community rather than in hospital. The 1983 Act allows such patients to be made the subject of what are known as 'guardianship' orders (s7(2) Mental Health Act 1983). A person of 16 years or over may be received into guardianship if s/he is suffering from mental disorder, i.e. mental illness, severe mental impairment, psychopathic disorder or mental impairment and the disorder is of a nature or degree warranting the use of guardianship and that it is in the interests of the patient or for the protection of others that guardianship powers be used. The guardian may be the local social services authority or other named person. An application for admission to guardianship may be made by an approved social worker or by the patient's nearest relative (s11(1)) and must contain the recommendation of two doctors. A clinical description of the patient's mental condition must be given and it must be explained why the patient cannot be appropriately cared for without the powers of guardianship.

One criticism made of the powers of guardianship has been that they are limited in scope. A patient may be required to live at a place specified by the guardian, and required to attend for treatment, occupation, education or training (s8). In addition, the order may require that a doctor or approved social worker be given access to the patient at his or her residence (s8). But a patient cannot be compelled to receive treatment. It appears that in practice these powers were rarely used (Gunn, 1986).

If a patient detained under section 3 is then released into the community s/he may be required, as a condition of discharge, to continue taking medication. But section 3 cannot be used to admit a patient with the aim of requiring him or her to receive medication and then releasing that patient into the community (*R* v. *Hallstrom exp W* [1986] QB 1090).

Some argued that patients were being released into the community but that there were inadequate powers for regulating their care, and thus patients would enter into a cycle of admission treatment and discharge followed by readmission. Concern as to this 'revolving door' led to the issue being considered by a House of Lords Select Committee in their 5th report (1992-93) and this was followed by a Department of Health Inquiry (DOH, 1993). The results of many of the recommendations for reform are to be found in the Mental Health (Patients in the Community) Act 1995. This legislation provides a new regime for supervision in the community of persons who have been released from detention (Mental Health Act 1983 s25A-H). The patient's responsible medical officer makes an application for supervision to the health authority which is to have responsibility for providing the patient with aftercare facilities (s25(A)s). The responsible medical officer (RMO) must be satisfied that supervision is justified on the basis of risk of harm to the patient or risk to the safety of others. In making this assessment the RMO should take into account the patient's views and those of persons who will be professionally concerned with the after care and others such as relatives who may be caring for the patient in the community (s25B). Once in the community the patient is under the care of a supervisor. As with guardianship the patient can be required to live in a particular place. The patients can be compelled to attend for treatment, but cannot be compelled to receive treatment (s25D). However, unlike guardianship, if the patient refuses treatment this may lead to his or her condition being reviewed to see whether readmission is necessary. Supervision under this power is for an initial period of 6 months with the possibility of renewal for a further 6 months. It may be ended at any time by the responsible medical officer after undertaking consultation (s25H(1)–(3)). This measure considerably strengthens the power to treat in the community.

Monitoring care - the role of the Mental Health Act Commission

The Mental Health Act Commission was established under the Mental Health Act 1983 (s120(1))(Bingley, 1995). The Commissioners are drawn from medical practitioners and others, such as social workers, academics, psychologists and lawyers. The Commission has the task of monitoring care given under the Act. The special hospitals are visited by the commissioners on a regular basis. They also visit other NHS hospitals and mental nursing homes which are registered to receive detained patients. They undertake periodic reviews of situations in which treatments have been authorised by the second opinion approved doctor. Where a nurse becomes concerned as to the regime at a mental health hospital and believes that her or his concerns have not been adequately addressed within the complaints structure available for hospital staff, then the Mental Health Act Commissioners provide one avenue through which s/he can address concerns as to standards of patient care (*Guidance to Staff on Dealings with Press and Media* (1993)) and they can also investigate complaints from patients (s120(1)(b) Mental Health Act 1983). They have the power to visit and interview detained patients. They can require the production of and inspection of records relating to detained patients.

The Commissioners may also make visits without giving advance warning if there is particular concern regarding patients. An example of this was a 'dawn raid' undertaken on 21 November 1996 on 31 acute psychiatric hospitals in England and Wales by the Mental Health Act Commission and the Sainsbury Centre for Mental Health. These raids led to a report which noted difficulties facing staff nursing and the mentally ill and the fact that staff appeared to be demotivated and that there were breakdowns in communication between staff and patients. The report noted that there were on average 80 patients for every 100 beds, which left little room for manoeuvre. The Commission monitors the implementation of the Mental Health Act Code of Practice.

The Commission publishes a biennial report which is laid before Parliament. It also publishes *Practice Notes*. Other functions include the appointment of second opinion doctors. The Mental Health Act Commission is itself accountable to the Secretary of State and to Parliament as a Special Health Authority.

References

Bate, P. (1994) 'Children on secure psychiatric units: out of sight out of mind.' *Journal of Child Law*, 131.

Bingley, W. (1995) 'The Mental Health Act Commission.' *Health Director*, 14.

Department of Health (1993) *Legal Powers of the Care of Mentally Ill People in the Community*. DOH, London.

Department of Health (1993) *Guidance for Staff on Relations with the Public and the Media.* (DOH), London.

Dimond, B. and Barker, F. (1996) *Mental Health Law for Nurses*. Blackwell Scientific, Oxford.

Fennell, P. (1994) 'Statutory authority to treat.' *Medical Law Review*, **2**, 30.

Gunn, M.J. (1986) 'Mental Health Act guardianship: where now?' *Journal of Social Welfare Law*, 144.

Gunn, M.J. (1994) 'Mental health nursing law.' in *Nursing Law and Ethics* (eds J. Tingle and A. Cribb). Blackwells, Oxford.

Hoggett, B. (1996) *Mental Health Law*, 4th edn. Sweet and Maxwell, London.

Law Commission (1995) *Mental Incapacity.* Law Com. Report No. 231. HMSO, London.

UKCC (1996) *Guidelines for Professional Practice*. United Kingdom Central Council for Nursing, Midwifery and Health Visiting, London.

Unsworth, C. (1987) *The Politics of Mental Health Legislation.* Clarendon Press, Oxford, p. 332.

Further reading

Brazier, M. and Bridge, C. (1996) 'Coercion or caring: analysing adolescent autonomy.' *Legal Studies*, **16**, 84.

Grubb, A. (ed.) (1993) 'Treatment decision: keeping it in the family.' In *Choices and Decisions in Health Care*. Wiley, Chichester.

McHale, J. and Fox, M. with Murphy, J. (1997) *Health Care Law Text and Materials*. Sweet and Maxwell, London, Chapters 7 and 9.

Chapter 7

Confidentiality and access to health care records

Jean McHale

Introduction

Confidentiality has long been emphasised in nursing practice. The Nightingale oath provided that:

> '...every nurse should be one who is to be depended upon, in other words, capable of being a 'confidential' nurse...she must be no gossip; no vain talker; she should never answer questions about her sick except to those who have a right to ask them; she must, I need not say be strictly sober and honest; but more than this, she must be a religious and devoted woman; she must have a respect for her calling.' (Nightingale, 1895)

It is still a fundamental part of nursing today. But as health care has grown in sophistication and complexity, so the boundaries of confidentiality have become increasingly difficult to define. Instead of receiving treatment all their life from one doctor, today patients are usually cared for in a group practice. During their time with that practice they may be seen by many different doctors and nurses. If they are given care in hospital the number of persons treating them will be considerably larger. The difficulty in maintaining confidentiality was graphically illustrated by Marc Siegler, a US physician and academic (Siegler, 1987). One of Siegler's patients threatened to leave hospital if he was not told just how many people did have access to his medical records. Siegler went away and came back with a figure of some 75 people - doctors, nurses, etc., who had legitimate access to his medical records; that did not include, of course, those who might have obtained unauthorised access. This patient was receiving relatively straightforward case of treatment. It is perhaps no wonder that, after being told this, the patient retorted, 'Perhaps you could explain just what you mean by confidentiality?'

This chapter examines the nurse's obligation to maintain her or his patient's confidence. (Difficulties relating to disclosure of the health care professional's own medical information to patients are examined in a later chapter.) The first part examines the general obligation of patient confidentiality; the second considers those situations in which health care information may be disclosed. Then the problems facing nurses are discussed when there are conflicts between maintaining patient confidentiality and upholding standards of care. Finally, safeguards for the confidentiality of health care records are discussed, and on what basis a patient may obtain access to such records.

General obligations

The nurse has an obligation to keep patient information confidential. This obligation covers both information disclosed to her or him directly and information which s/he obtains from other health care professionals when treating the patient. The obligation of confidentiality is contained in the nurse's professional ethical code. The United Kingdom Central Council for Nursing, Midwifery and Health Visiting code (UKCC, 1993i) provides that the nurse must:

> 'protect all confidential information concerning patients and clients obtained in the course of professional practice and make disclosures only with consent, where required by the order of the court or where you can justify disclosure in the wider public interest.'

The extent of this obligation is now set out in the new UKCC guidance document (UKCC, 1996). Secondly, the nurse's contract of employment requires her or him to keep patient information confidential. Unauthorised disclosure may lead the nurse to be disciplined by her or his professional body or to be dismissed by the employer. Thirdly, where information has been disclosed in breach of an obligation of confidence legal proceedings may follow, such as an injunction being obtained to stop further publication of the confidential information. For example, in *X* v. *Y* ([1988] 2 All ER 648) the medical records of two general practitioners who had developed AIDS were disclosed in a national newspaper. The court issued an injunction to stop further publication of the records. To bring legal proceedings for breach of confidence the patient must show that a duty of confidence, either express or implied, has arisen, that the information was given in confidence and that disclosure was made in breach of that duty (*Att. Gen* v. *Guardian Newspaper* (No 2) [1988] 3 All ER 545). A duty of confidence would be implied in a situation in which a patient discloses information to a nurse because of her or his status as a nurse.

The nurse is thus obliged in both law and professional practice to keep the patient's confidence. But this obligation is not regarded as absolute - in some situations the nurse may legitimately break confidence. In addition, the nurse may be required to break confidentiality by court order or by specific statutory provision. These issues will be examined further below.

Children and confidentiality

What right does a child patient have to confidentiality? It is ludicrous to suggest that a nurse shouldn't discuss a toddler's illness with the child's mother. But, children grow and begin to express the wish to control aspects of their own lives. If a 14-year-old girl approaches a school nurse and asks for advice regarding contraceptive treatment, what should the nurse do?

In *Gillick* v. *West Norfolk and Wisbech AHA* ([1986] AC 150) Mrs Victoria Gillick sought an assurance from her local health authority that her daughter would not be given advice concerning contraception/abortion or receive treatment without her consent. The authority refused to give the assurance and Mrs Gillick went to court and asked for a declaration that the authority's decision and the guidance of the DHSS on which the authority's refusal was based were unlawful. She was unsuccessful in her application. In the House of Lords it was said that the child is able to consent to medical treatment where she has sufficient maturity to do so.

While the *Gillick* case was primarily concerned with consent to treatment, nevertheless it appears to be the case that this approach would be followed in relation to confidentiality (Montgomery 1987; Grubb and Pearl 1987). A health professional should not usually disclose information in the case of a *Gillick* competent child to a third party without that child's consent. This does give rise to some difficult issues as to whether a child has sufficient competence to consent (see Chapter 6). Where the child patient is very young, disclosure of information to the parents may be an integral part of the child's care. Nevertheless, the nurse should think long and hard before s/he decides to disclose a child's medical information without the child's consent.

The incompetent patient

The extent to which an obligation of confidence is owed to a patient who is permanently incompetent, such as a mentally handicapped patient, is unclear. In the absence of decided authority it is submitted that it is likely that the general position taken by the House of Lords in the context of consent to treatment in the case of *Re F* ([1990] 1 AC 1) should be followed and that information may be disclosed only where it is in that patient's best interests to do so.

After the patient's death

The obligation of confidentiality continues after the patient's death. When Lord Moran, the physician of Winston Churchill, published a book which discussed the decline of the great war leader (*Churchill - The Struggle for Survival*) he was roundly condemned by his contemporaries. As Mason and McCall Smith (1994i) note, confidentiality after death is something which may be of particular importance in the age of AIDS. But while maintenance of confidentiality after death may be part of the professional's ethical obligation, it is less certain whether legal proceedings could be brought in such circumstances. An action for libel and slander cannot be brought after the death of the person who has been defamed. It has been suggested that a court might reject a claim of breach of confidence brought after the patient's death on the basis that the obligation only existed during that patient's lifetime (Kennedy and Grubb, 1994i).

Grounds for disclosure

Patient care would be impossible unless some disclosure of information was made. Certain recognised exceptions do exist. Nevertheless, the nurse should be aware that all disclosures should be carefully justified.

Disclosing with consent

Disclosure is both lawful and complies with professional ethical codes if the patient has given consent to the information being passed on. Such consent must be freely and fully given. However, in practice this may not always be the case. As Mason and McCall Smith (1994ii) comment:

> 'What patient at a teaching hospital out-patients department is likely to refuse when the consultant asks 'You don't mind these young doctors being present, don't you?' - the pressures are virtually irresistible and truly autonomous consent is impossible.'

It can be argued that when a patient who enters hospital s/he impliedly consents to such information as is necessary for her or his treatment being passed to other health care practitioners. But consent to disclosure should not always be presumed. The UKCC (1996i) now states in the document *Guidelines for Professional Practice* that:

> 'It is impractical to obtain the consent of patient or client every time you need to share information with other health professionals or other staff involved in the health care of that patient or client. What is important is that the patient or client understands that some information may be made available to others involved in the delivery of their care. However, the patient or client must know who the information would be shared with.'

As the Department of Health (1996) has stated in its guidance:

> 'All NHS bodies must have an active policy for informing patients of the kind of purposes for which information about them is collected and the categories of people or organisations to which information may need to be passed.'

The nurse must ensure that from the onset of care the patient is aware that some information may be disclosed to third parties who are involved in her or his care. Where disclosure is necessary then information should be disclosed on a 'need to know' basis. The Department of Health (1996i) has suggested that this includes NHS purposes where 'the recipient needs the information because he or she is or may be concerned with the patient's care or treatment (or that of another patient whose health may be affected by the condition of the original patient, such as a blood or organ donor)'.

Public interest exception

The courts have held that in some situations disclosure of confidential information is justifiable in the public interest. The UKCC code also recognises a public interest exception. What amounts to disclosure in the public interest by a health care professional was examined by the courts in *W* v. *Egdell* ([1990] ChD 359). A breach of confidence action was brought against a psychiatrist. He had been commissioned by W's solicitors to make a medical report on W's fitness for discharge from the secure hospital where he had been detained after he was convicted of manslaughter 8 years previously. The report was highly unfavourable to W and W's solicitors withdrew their application to a Mental Health Review Tribunal. Dr Egdell told the solicitors that he believed that a copy of the report should be put on W's hospital file. The solicitors disagreed. Dr Egdell himself sent a copy to the hospital. This fact emerged at a subsequent Mental Health Review Tribunal hearing and an action for breach of confidence was brought against Dr Egdell by W.

The case was first heard in the High Court. Scott J. rejected the claim that Dr Edgell was wrong to have disclosed the information. He noted that W was not an ordinary member of the public. In his opinion the doctor owed a duty not only to W but also to the public. This required him to place before the proper authorities the result of his examination of W. He placed weight upon the fact that while in detention W had been seen by a number of psychiatrists. Each of these owed him a duty of confidence such that they could not, for example, sell the information to a newspaper, but, at the same time the reports compiled about W were on file and were available to the Home Office. In the view of Scott J. the fact that these reports were on file had not inhibited W in his dealings with these psychiatrists. He did not believe that the report of Dr Egdell should be treated any differently.

W appealed to the Court of Appeal where his appeal was rejected. Sir Stephen Brown was broadly in agreement with the first instance decision. Disclosure of the information was in the public interest in ensuring the safety of the public as a whole. The effect of suppressing the material contained in the report would have been to deprive both the hospital and the Secretary of State of vital information. The other judge to deliver a full judgment in this case, Bingham J., was more cautious. He stressed that a patient such as W who was held under a restriction order had a very great need for recourse to a professional advisor who is independent and discreet. The confidentiality of such patients should only be broken if needed on the basis of the doctor's duty to society. On the facts of this particular case, Bingham J. held that disclosure had been justified. The decisive facts were that:

> 'Where a man has committed multiple killings under the disability of serious mental illness, decisions which may lead directly or indirectly to his release from hospital should not be made unless a responsible authority is able to make an informed judgment that the risk of repetition is so small as to be acceptable.'

W v. *Egdell* clearly illustrates that confidentiality in law is far from an absolute obligation. In each case the court will balance the public interest in ensuring confidentiality against the public interest in disclosure. In determining public interest the courts will make reference to the guidelines set out by the health care professionals. Nurses are given some guidance as to circumstances that may justify disclosure in the public interest by the UKCC (1996ii) in its recent document *Guidelines for Professional Practice.* This states that:

> 'The public interest means the interests of an individual, or groups of individuals or of society as a whole, and would, for example, cover matters such as serious crime, child abuse, drug trafficking or other activities which place others at serious risk.'

It is fairly certain that disclosure of the fact that your patient has a mental illness which makes him a potential danger to the community to the appropriate authorities will be held to be in the public interest. Similarly, if a nurse was told of child abuse and s/he discloses this information to an agency such as the NSPCC it is likely that a court would hold that the disclosure was in the public interest. Nevertheless, there are other situations in which it is not clear whether the public interest justifies disclosure. A nurse who discovers that a patient has committed shoplifting offences should hesitate long before disclosing that fact. Again, the nurse may face a dilemma if a patient tells her or him that he knows the identity of the person who stabbed him but does not want the nurse to give this information to the police because the patient is frightened of retaliation from a gang of thugs. In such a situation the nurse should attempt to persuade the patient to approach the police himself.

What if a patient who is diagnosed as HIV positive refuses to tell his wife? Should the nurse or any other health care professional inform the man's wife? The man may be frightened that his marriage would break up if his wife is told. The General Medical Council has advised doctors that disclosure may be justifiable if there is a serious and identifiable risk to a specific individual (GMC, 1995). The legal position here is unclear but it is suggested that if disclosure did take place a court would be prepared to hold that the breach of confidence was in the public interest.

Police enquiries

A police constable comes into hospital reception. He wants to ask questions of the ward sister and to search through a particular patient's medical records. Can he do this? Firstly, if the ward sister is asked questions she is under no obligation to answer them. In English law there is no general obligation placed upon any citizen to answer questions put to them by the police (*Rice* v. *Connolly* [1966] 2QB416) although if a defendant keeps silent there is a possibility that an adverse inference may be drawn regarding the decision to keep silent (Criminal Justice Act 1994). There are also some exceptional situations in which disclosure is required by statute. For example, under the Prevention of Terrorism (Temporary Provisions) Act 1989, a person can be prosecuted if s/he withholds information relating to acts of terrorism (s18). Secondly, the police have no automatic right to demand access to a patient's records. Access to medical records by police conducting enquiries is regulated by statute. Usually, before the police may examine a patient's medical records they must obtain a warrant under the Police and Criminal Evidence Act 1984 (PACE) (s9-s11 and schedule 1). Before a police constable can gain access to premises such as a doctor's surgery or a hospital in order to search for information such as medical records/samples of human tissue, or tissue fluid taken for the purpose of diagnosis/medical treatment or held in confidence, s/he must apply to a circuit judge for a warrant. The police must show that there is a reasonable belief that the information needed is contained on the premises and that prior to the 1984 Act a statute existed under which the police could have obtained the information. There is, however, no duty upon the police when applying for a warrant to inform the person whose confidential information is sought about the application. Only the person who is holding the information - in the case of hospital medical records an administrator - must be told. It is submitted that this is undesirable and that the patient should, wherever possible, have a voice at the hearing. It appears that the courts have been prepared to scrutinise carefully applications for medical records. For example, in *R* v. *Cardiff Crown Court ex parte Kellam* (1993) 16 BMCR 76, the court refused to allow police who were investigating a murder of a mental patient to obtain access to records of admission, discharge and leave of patients at the hospital.

In practice if, for example, the police ask a nurse for access to medical records, the UKCC (1996iii) advises that 'it may be appropriate to involve senior staff if you do not feel that you are able to deal with the situation alone'.

Civil law proceedings

If a patient is injured due to what s/he claims is negligent treatment, the patient will need to obtain evidence in the form of, for example, medical reports to establish a case. The patient's lawyers will ask for access to the records. If this is refused, then an application must be made to the court under the Administration of Justice Act 1970 for disclosure of documents. Section 32 makes particular reference to records which are sought in a personal injury action. Here, the court can order that reports are made available to the applicant, to his or her legal advisor or, if the applicant does not have a legal advisor, to his or her medical advisors (s33 and s34 Supreme Court Act 1981). As has been commented (Mason and McCall Smith, 1994i):

> '...the court can deal with problems of confidentiality relating to irrelevant conditions - such as a past history of a sexually transmitted disease - by limiting disclosure to the other side's medical advisors who must respect confidentiality save where litigation is affected.'

In addition, disclosure of expert reports should be made at the pre-hearing stage (*Naylor* v. *Preston AHA* [1987] 2 All ER 353). There are, however, exceptions to the general requirements of disclosure. For example, communications between a plaintiff and his or her lawyer are usually not required to be disclosed. Such communications are covered by what is known as 'legal professional privilege' (for discussion of the operation of the trial process see Chapter 10).

Evidence in court

If a nurse is summoned as a witness in court case s/he must give evidence. There is no special rule of evidence – no evidential 'privilege' which would entitle the nurse to refuse to testify (McHale, 1993; *Duchess of Kingston's case* (1776) 20 State Trials 355). If the nurse refuses to disclose any information in response to any question put to her or him, then a judge may find the nurse in contempt of court and may ultimately send the nurse to prison.

Public health disclosure requirements

In some situations, disclosure of medical information is required by statute as a public health measure in order to limit the spread of certain diseases. Notifiable diseases include cholera, plague, smallpox, typhus, and rabies (s11 Public Health (Control of Disease) Act 1984). Where a registered medical practitioner becomes aware or suspects that a patient s/he is attending is suffering from such an illness, the practitioner must notify the local authority of the patient's name, age, sex, the disease from which the patient is suffering and the date of onset of the disease.

Release of information without patient's permission

The UKCC (1996iv) in its document *Guidelines for Professional Practice* suggests that before information is disclosed without a patient's consent, the nurse should consult with her or his colleagues, and it may be appropriate to consult an organisation such as the UKCC. If it is decided to disclose the UKCC suggests that the nurse should record the reasons for disclosure, and thus the justification for any action taken, in the appropriate record or in a special note in a separate file.

Unauthorised disclosures

Unauthorised disclosures should be minimised. It is unethical to discuss a patient's case outside the clinical setting with friends, or discuss a case with colleagues in public where one may be overheard. In hospital, records should never be left lying around where unauthorised persons may read them. It is important to ensure that safeguards exist against disclosure, particularly where a patient is, for example, suffering from AIDS. A minimal number of clinical staff necessary to facilitate that patient's care should be informed that the patient is HIV positive. Nurses have also been advised by the RCN to avoid giving information over the phone because of the problem of verifying the identity of the caller and also the risk of being overheard (RCN, 1991).

Computerised medical records

Most patient records are now held on computer. Holding data on computer enables easy passage of data through the NHS family. However there is always a danger that hackers may enter the system and abuse the data. As the UKCC emphasises in its *Guidelines*, access to computer systems must be carefully controlled (UKCC, 1996v). Unauthorised access may lead to a prosecution under the Computer Misuse Act 1990.

Occupational health context

Nurses employed by organisations other than the NHS may face some very difficult disclosure dilemmas. Take, for example, the occupational health nurse employed by a large industrial firm. The nurse owes a duty to the employer, but at the same time as a caring professional s/he is bound by professional ethical code. If the nurse intends that the information given by the patient s/he is treating should be disclosed to the employer, then the nurse must make this clear to the patient before undertaking the consultation.

Legal obligation to break confidence?

Can the nurse ever be required to disclose information and be held liable in negligence if s/he does not do so? What if a patient tells a nurse of his or her wish to harm another person; should that nurse warn the person who might be in danger? This issue arose in the United States in the case of *Tarasoff* v. *Regents of the University of California* ([1976] 551 P 2d 334).

Poddar, a university student, sought out patient care in a psychiatric hospital. He was suffering from deep depression as a result of being rejected by one Miss Tarasoff with whom he had fallen in love. He told a psychologist at the hospital of his intention to kill Miss Tarasoff. After discussions with psychiatrists, the psychologist decided that Podder should be detained in a mental hospital. He told the campus police, who detained Poddar but later released him when he appeared to be rational. Two months after the consultation with the psychologist, Poddar killed Miss Tarasoff. The majority in the Californian Supreme Court held that the therapist was under a duty to warn both victim and victim's family and was liable for his failure to do so.

The *Tarasoff* case led to an outcry from psychiatric associations in the United States. The court reconsidered its decision some 18 months later. It modified the duty from one to warn the victim to one of exercising reasonable care for the victim's protection and to take steps reasonably necessary in the circumstances. In a memorable phrase it was said that the 'protective privilege ends when the public peril begins'.

There are echoes of *Tarasoff* in the judgment of Scott J. in the English case of *W* v. *Egdell*, a judgment which received the approval of Sir Stephen Brown in the Court of Appeal. Scott J. held that:

> 'In my view as a doctor called upon as Dr Egdell was to examine a patient owes a duty not only to his patient, but also to the public. His duty to the public would require him, in my opinion, to place before the proper authorities the results of his examination if, in his opinion, the public interest so requires.'

What did Scott J. mean here by the duty to disclose? Will a court in future be prepared to find that a health care professional owes a duty of care to the person his patient claims that he is going to kill or seriously injure? At present it seems unlikely that an English court would impose such an obligation. The courts have been unwilling in the past to extend the scope of liability imposed upon third parties (*Smith* v. *Littlewood* [1987] 1 All ER 710). Any obligation to disclose may limit an individual's privacy if practitioners feel that they must go ahead and disclose to avoid being sued in negligence.

Negotiated confidentiality

Confidentiality is an important obligation but determining the boundaries may prove problematic, as has been seen. One suggestion which has been advanced is that the practice of negotiated confidentiality could be adopted (Sieghart, 1982; Thompson, 1979). Practitioner and patient discuss the extent to which patient information should remain confidential. They negotiate as to what information may be disclosed and what information may not. One major advantage is that negotiation removes much uncertainty. Both parties know the ground rules for disclosure. However, such an approach is not without difficulties. It involves effort and understanding. There is also the danger that when the negotiations were undertaken some criteria relating to disclosure had not been envisaged. Negotiation is also time consuming and it may not be a practical prospect in many situations.

Confidentiality – specific obligations

In addition to the general obligations spelt out above, certain specific obligations of confidentiality have been imposed by statute.

Human Fertilisation and Embryology Act 1990

Few statutes expressly require patient confidentiality to be maintained. One exception is the Human Fertilisation and Embryology Act 1990. This Act regulates the provision of new reproductive technology services. Information relating to infertility treatment is particularly sensitive. Section 33 of the 1990 Act places a statutory ban upon the disclosure of information concerning gamete donors and patients receiving treatment under the Act. Unauthorised disclosure of such information by health care professionals and others has been made a criminal offence (1990 Act s40(1)(5)).

There are certain exceptions to the general obligation. The clinician at the *in vitro* fertility (IVF) unit may disclose information where the patient has consented to that disclosure to a specific person (1990 Act s33 (6B) or where it is necessary to disclose the information to a person who 'needs to know' for the purposes of treating the patient or where a medical emergency has arisen or in connection with clinical or accounts audit (1990 Act s33(6c)). This statutory exception is itself the source of some controversy, particularly in view of the fact that it is now routine practice in IVF clinics to require patients to take HIV tests. It is questionable whether a patient's GP is entitled to know the fact that his patient has tested HIV positive. This is another instance in which the 'need to know' should be tightly interpreted.

Venereal disease

Legislation restricting disclosure of patient information also exists in the area of venereal diseases. The National Health Service Venereal Disease Regulations (SI 1974 No. 29) provide that Health Authorities should take all necessary steps to ensure that identifiable information relating to persons being treated for sexually transmitted diseases should not be disclosed. Such information may be disclosed where this is for the purpose of communicating the information to a doctor caring for the patient, or to a person working under the direction of that doctor to treat that condition or to prevent its spread.

Conflicts between confidentiality and the need to uphold standards of care

The UKCC code requires the nurse to report circumstances in which the standard of care given has fallen below levels which are acceptable:

> 'As a registered nurse, midwife and health visitor you are personally accountable for your practice and, in the exercise of your professional accountability, must :
>
> 11. report to an appropriate person or authority having regard to the physical, psychological and social effects on patients and clients any circumstances in the environment of care which could jeopardise safe standards of practice;
> 12. report to an appropriate person or authority any circumstances in which safe and appropriate care for patients and clients cannot be provided;
> 13. report to an appropriate person or authority where it appears that the health and safety of colleagues is at risk, as such circumstances may compromise standards of practice and care.'

The UKCC notes in the document *Guidelines for Professional Practice* that these are a statement of the minimum action to be taken (UKCC, 1996vi) and that:

> 'You must not be deterred from reporting your concerns, even if you believe that resources are not available or that no action will be taken. You should make your report, verbally and/or in writing, and where available, follow local procedures. The manager (who may also be registered with us) should assess the report and communicate it to senior managers where appropriate. (UKCC, 1996vii)'

As commented, this record may be of importance if subsequent action is taken against the nurse and s/he claims that the actions which s/he took were affected by the fact that there were inadequate resources.

There may be instances in which the obligation of confidentiality owed by nurse to patient may conflict with the nurse's belief that standards of patient care had fallen. This problem arose in the case of Graham Pink. Pink was a charge nurse who believed that standards of hospital services provided to his elderly patients were unsatisfactory. Although he complained within the management structure, he did not believe that his complaints had been addressed. He was concerned about:

> 'avoidable injuries to patients (including a death); important observations for people on blood transfusions not carried out; patients offered a wash once a day...'(Letter to the chairman of Stockport Health Authority, *The Guardian*, 9 July 1991)'

Thus, as a result of obtaining no response to his complaints, Pink made the decision to go public about his concerns: he wrote letters to *The*

Guardian newspaper; he gave an interview to a local paper. The health authority brought disciplinary proceedings against him on the basis of breach of patient confidentiality. Although the article did not name patients, relatives claimed that a patient could be identified from details of his case given in the press report. Pink was also charged with not reporting an incident in which a patient fell out of bed. At the disciplinary hearing the allegations were upheld against Pink and when he refused to transfer to a post of community nurse he was dismissed (*The Guardian*, 18 Sept 1991).

As the Pink case shows the threat of dismissal for breach of confidentiality is a very real one. Pink challenged his dismissal at an industrial tribunal. A claim can be brought before a tribunal for unlawful dismissal on the grounds that the dismissal was unfair (s98 Employment Rights Act 1996). The tribunal decides whether the action taken by the employer was reasonable and assesses her or his dismissal on the balance of competing equities. There is, however, no general protection in employment law given to those employees who believe that they have disclosed in the public interest. Pink's case was ultimately settled before any final decision was made by the tribunal.

If a nurse does not take action about what s/he regards as undesirably low standards then the nurse runs the risk of being disciplined by the UKCC. The UKCC code was claimed in his defence by Graham Pink. However, as Pink discovered, simply acting in accordance with the UKCC code is by itself no defence should the employee's action breach the duty of employment.

The Government issued a document providing guidance for staff who are considering making complaints about what they regard as being poor standards of care (DOH, 1993). Firstly, the guidelines stress that procedures should be set up to deal with staff grievances. Informal procedures should be available but where these do not lead to a satisfactory resolution there should be formal procedures in existence to enable concerns to be ventilated. The formal complaints should be made either up the line management chain or to a designated officer who may be the person designated to receive patient complaints. This has been criticised in that staff may be frightened to make such a reference because of the consequences for their own careers if they are regarded as being troublemakers. As Public Concern at Work commented in relation to the draft guidelines:

> 'To require a concerned member of staff to confront his or her line manager on their judgment or priorities in this way is unlikely to be productive or conducive for a good working environment. Only the most exceptional manager would not, in such a situation want to pull rank over the staff member concerned. (McHale, 1994)'

The guidelines distinguish between those health care professionals who are in a direct line management relationship and others not in such a relationship, such as consultants. In relation to the latter it is suggested that they discuss their concerns with relevant colleagues and then take the matter up directly with the general manager or chief executive. This difference in approach may be seen as undesirable and indeed as divisive.

The guidelines suggest that if complaints are made to a designated officer and the matter is not resolved then the issue should be referred to the chairman of the authority or trust for action to be taken. There is no external right of appeal, the highest level of appeal being within the existing management framework. The guidelines state that in some situations, health care professionals may wish to consult with outside agencies. For example, where a nurse is concerned about the welfare of a patient detained under the Mental Health Act 1983 s/he may decide to take the complaint to the Mental Health Act Commission (see page 97 above).

The guidelines make reference to the fact that health professionals may raise concerns with the Health Service Commissioner (the Ombudsman). While at present the Commissioner may not receive general complaints from hospital staff concerning standards, nevertheless he has indicated that he is willing to receive complaints from staff if they are made on behalf of an individual patient, the patient himself is unable to complain, and there is no other person who could claim on the patient's behalf. In his 1991-92 report, the Commissioner commented that he had undertaken an investigation of a complaint brought by a member of staff indicating that the level of care which a patient was receiving was inadequate (Health Service Commissioner, 1992). Access to the Commissioner may indeed be a helpful way of ventilating staff concerns. However, the Commissioner's office has only limited resources and it may take a certain amount of time to process a claim.

One welcome provision of the guidelines is the right to consult a professional agency such as a trade union or other representative agency (DOH 1993 clause 23). Health care professionals may also of course raise their concerns with their MP. It is only at the very end of the guidelines that the question of disclosure to the media itself is considered. Such disclosure is regarded as a matter of last resort and should the nurse make the decision to 'go public', as did Graham Pink, then the guidelines remind the nurse that s/he is at risk of disciplinary proceedings. The guidelines refer to the duty of confidentiality to preserve patient information and the duty of confidentiality and loyalty to the employer (DOH 1993 clauses 8 and 9). Should a nurse find the internal mechanisms inadequate for dealing with concerns then s/he is left with the choice of going public, with the risk of legal and disciplinary proceedings should s/he do so.

The guidelines met considerable opposition when they were originally published. Reg Pyne, former Assistant Registrar at the UKCC, called them 'seriously flawed' and 'oppressive' (Turner, 1994). While their publication can in one respect be regarded as an important step recognising that an important issue should be addressed nevertheless, as was suggested above, in many ways they may be regarded as unsatisfactory. A number of proposals have been made for their reform. Geoffrey Hunt, in his concluding chapter to a collection of essays on 'whistleblowing', makes a number of proposals (Hunt, 1994). First, there needs to be a change in the culture ensuring that there is greater receptivity to complaints in the workplace. This may be fostered by a code of ethics for health service managers. Hunt proposes the establishment of a procedure for ethical audit of all those procedures which maintain public accountability of managers and employees.

A more radical approach would be to create some form of hospital standards organisation which would perhaps accredit hospitals. There is already a movement towards accreditation in this country through the Kings Fund Hospital Accreditation Scheme (Scrivens, 1995). Extension of this scheme could be linked to a staff complaints system. Attempts have also been made to introduce legislation protecting those who 'blow the whistle' in the public interest, notably by Maurice Franklin MP in 1995. In the USA, whistleblowing legislation has been enacted but it has had a checkered existence (McHale, 1994). It appears that people are frequently afraid to use the statutes; while they may, for example, win a case in employment law they are unlikely to be reinstated to their job. One option would be to reform employment law to protect those dismissed on the basis of public interest. But this would still mean that an industrial tribunal would have to assess whether dismissal for breach of confidence was in the public interest. Ultimately the most important factor may be change in the organisational culture to promote trust.

Health care records - allowing patient access

Record keeping is an important part of nursing practice. Principles of record keeping in general are examined in the section on General obligations above. In this section, the extent to which patients may access their own records is considered, and the particular obligations placed upon the nurse to maintain the security of these records against unauthorised disclosure to third parties. The 1980s saw a dramatic shift in the policy of allowing patients access to their medical records. In the past, there was considerable opposition to patient access. There were several reasons for this. Firstly, it was argued that the patient would have difficulty in understanding the records because they may have been compiled using technical terms or medical shorthand. Secondly, if health care professionals knew that a patient could gain access, they would not be so candid in their comments when compiling the records. Thirdly, it was argued that to allow access may be against the patient's interests because records may contain information which had been deliberately kept from the patient, for example showing a terminal prognosis. But these arguments met with criticism. It was claimed that access to records is a fundamental part of patient autonomy and the denial of access in the patient's best interests is a paternalistic approach. It was said that a blanket ban was wrong because, while some patients might be unable to cope with the information, this did not mean that all patients were unable to cope. If health care records were incomprehensible to patients this was not a basis for denying access; rather, it should be ensured that the records are comprehensible.

Data Protection Act 1984

Parliament has now intervened and access to health care records is regulated by statute. A right of access was first granted to health care records held on computer by the Data Protection Act 1984. A person whose data are held on computer (the data subject) may request to see his or her records from the holder of the computerised medical record (the data user) (s21). If s/he believes that the records are erroneous, s/he can apply for the records to be amended. If a patient has suffered distress or damage from the inaccurate data, s/he has a right to claim compensation (s22(1)(4)). If a patient is incapable, due to mental disorder, of making his or her own application a request can be made on the patient's behalf (s21(9)). Children may apply to see their own records if they are regarded as having sufficient maturity to do so. However, the Act does not give parents a right to see their child's medical records. This creates an obvious problem in the case of a very young child. One solution suggested is that, as the Act allows the data user to make certain disclosures to third parties, information may be disclosed to the child's parents (Kennedy and Grubb, 1994iii).

Access To Medical Reports Act 1988

The Data Protection Act was followed by the Access to Medical Reports Act 1988, which granted a statutory right of access to reports compiled for the purposes of employment or insurance (s2). This right covers only those reports made by a person who has had clinical care of the patient, and would exclude a one-off examination specifically undertaken for the purposes of insurance by a clinician previously unknown to the patient. The patient who has requested that such a report be drawn up has the right to see the report. If the patient does not request the report it cannot be sent for 3 weeks (s4). If s/he believes it to be inaccurate, the patient may ask the doctor to amend it (s5). If the doctor refuses, then the patient can either refuse to allow the report to be sent to the employer or insurer, or can have his or her own comments added to the report.

Access To Health Records Act 1990

A general right of access to medical records was finally introduced by the Access to Health Records Act 1990 (NHS Executive, 1990). This Act gave patients, for the first time, a right to obtain certain manual records drawn up by health professionals. Access may be sought from a whole range of health professionals including nurses (s1(1)). In the case of general practice records, the application is usually made to the patient's GP. An application for access to NHS hospital records should be made to the appropriate health authority or NHS trust. Private patients should apply directly to the health professional (s1(2)). Parents or guardians can obtain access to records on behalf of their children. The child can obtain access him- or herself as long as s/he is capable of understanding the nature of the application for access (s4).The patient may be entitled to see the record or any part of it, or s/he may be entitled to see extracts from the record. The patient must be given an explanation of any terms within the record which may be intelligible without explanation (s3(2)). The patient is entitled to ask that a note be included in his or her records to the effect that s/he would not wish others to have access to the record after the patient's death (s4(3)).

The 1990 Access to Health Records Act does not apply to those records compiled prior to the Act coming into force on 1 November 1991. Claims to access records compiled prior to that date must be brought at common law. The courts have stated that while there is no automatic right under common law to obtain access to medical records, information may be disclosed by a health care professional exercising professional judgment (*R* v. *Mid Glamorgan FHSA ex parte Martin* [1995] 1 All ER 356).

While at present there is no general oversight over access to information held on manual records in the form of an officer such as the Data Protection Registrar, this now appears likely to change with the passage of a recent EU Directive governing data, including those stored manually (EU Directive 95/46/EC).

Limitations to rights of access

It must be emphasised that the rights of access to health information under the above pieces of legislation are not absolute. In all cases, information may be withheld if the information would cause serious harm to a patient's physical or mental state or that of another person (Data Protection Act) (Subject Access Modification (Health) Order 1987 SI No. 1903: Access to Medical Reports Act 1988 s17: Access to Health Records Act 1990 s5(1)). This clinical privilege needs to be exercised with considerable sensitivity if the rights of the patient are to be adequately protected. As Brazier (1992) notes:

> 'What should not be forgotten is that a patient who genuinely would rather not know what was wrong with him will never ask for access to his records.'

Another limitation upon access is that patients may, and it appears usually are, charged for access to their medical information. The Access to Health Records Act 1990 allows a patient to be charged a fee of up to £10 if the record has not been added to within the last 40 days. Where information concerns infertility treatment, this is governed by the Human

Fertilisation and Embryology Act 1990. Access to information by those born as a consequence of infertility services regulated under the 1990 Act is limited to those over 18 who have been given the opportunity of obtaining counselling (s31(3) 1990 Act).

Ensuring the security of records

The nurse must ensure that patient records are kept secure from unauthorised access. This is particularly important in view of the fact that so much information today is held on computer. The UKCC document *Guidelines for Professional Practice* emphasises the need to keep confidence. It states that:

> 'As far as computer-held records are concerned, you must be satisfied that as far as is possible, the methods you use for recording information are secure. You must also find out which categories of staff have access to records to which they are expected to contribute important personal and confidential information. Local procedures must include ways of checking whether a record is authentic where there is no written signature. All records must clearly indicate the identity of the person who made that record (UKCC, 1996viii).'

Unauthorised access to information held on computer may constitute a criminal offence under the Computer Misuse Act 1990 although there are certain exceptions in relation to a situation in which a person accidentally exceeds his or her permission.

Unauthorised disclosure of health information

There have been suggestions that if a practitioner goes ahead and discloses confidential information without the consent of that patient, the practitioner may be held liable in negligence for that disclosure. Carson and Montgomery (1990) give an example of a case in which a doctor was held to be liable in negligence for revealing to the husband of his patient the fact that he considered that she was paranoid. He had not told the patient directly because he thought that this would cause harm to the patient's mental state and to the doctor-patient relationship. It was held that the harm which took place was reasonably foreseeable in nature, even though the circumstances in which the husband revealed the information were not.

Should patients be allowed to retain their own records?

Health care records are usually held in hospitals, health centres or surgeries although certain trials have been conducted to ascertain the feasibility of patients being given their own records on 'smart cards' - small cards on which data are electronically stored and which may be accessed by a special machine. However, the fact that a patient is simply given a smart card by itself will not facilitate access to records, because access is dependent upon the patient having means to access the information on that card.

But if the general principle of patient access is accepted then why not allow patients to keep hold of their own records? There is, of course, the risk that patients would lose them, but studies undertaken seem to suggest that this is not the case (Gilhooley and McGhee, 1991) There are considerable advantages in patient-held records. For example, nurses would have immediate access to records if visiting patients at home; there would be no delay in transferring records when the patient moved GP; time would be saved in GPs' surgeries storing records; it would assist patients in correcting inaccuracies in records. It may also increase trust between patients and health care professionals. As the UKCC (1993ii) has stated:

> 'Patient or client held records help to emphasise and make clear the practitioner's responsibility to the patient or client by sharing any information held or assessments made and illustrate the involvement of the patient or client in their own care.'

However, as the UKCC notes, there are limitations to client held records because the health professional may want to include information to be withheld from a client. The UKCC (1996) suggests that in some situations, in view of the concerns of the health professional, a supplementary record should be created, for example in relation to such matters as child abuse.

Conclusions

Reforming the law

The present law concerning patient confidentiality can only be gleaned by reference to a number of disparate sources. The boundaries of disclosure for the nurse are unclear. In 1995 the British Medical Association produced a draft Bill on confidentiality. The Bill was the result of deliberations by a working party which included nursing input from the UKCC. A version of this Bill was introduced into the House of Lords by Lord Walton in 1996 and was given a second reading. This Bill applied to information relating to an individual's physical or mental health which is in the control of a health service body or qualified health professional. It set out the basis on which information could be lawfully disclosed and made unauthorised disclosure a criminal offence. It ultimately was unsuccessful and, at present, comprehensive legislation appears unlikely. Nonetheless, while clarification of the boundaries of disclosure is surely to be welcomed, ultimately the best safeguard of patient confidentiality is that of good professional norms.

References

Brazier, M. (1992) *Medicine, Patients and the Law*, 2nd edn. Penguin, Harmondsworth.
Carson, D. and Montgomery, J. (1990) *Nursing Law*. Macmillan, Basingstoke.
Department of Health (1993) *Guidance for Staff on Relations With the Public and the Media*. DOH, London.
Department of Health (1996) *The Protection and Use of Personal Health Information*. DOH, London.
General Medical Council *HIV and AIDS: the ethical considerations*. GMC, London.
Gilhooley, M. and McGhee, S.M. (1991) 'Medical records; practicalities and principles of patient possession.' *Journal of Medical Ethics*, **17**, 138.
Grubb, A. and Pearl, D. (1986) 'Medicine, Health, Family and the law.' *Family Law*, **101**.
Health Service Commissioner (1992) *Annual Report for 1991-92*. HMSO, London, HC 82.
Hunt, G. (ed.) (1994) *Whistleblowing in the Health Service*. Edward Arnold, London.
Kennedy, I. and Grubb, A. (1994) *Medical Law, Text With Materials*. Butterworths, London.
Kloss, D. (1994) *Occupational Health*, 2nd edn. Blackwell Scientific, Oxford.
Mason, J.K. and McCall Smith, R.A. (1994) *Law and Medical Ethics*, 4th edn. Butterworths, London, (i) p189 (ii) p168 (iii) p184.
McHale, J.V. (1993) *Medical Confidentiality and Legal Privilege*. Routledge, London.
McHale, J. (1994) 'Whistleblowing in the USA.' In *Whistleblowing in the Health Services* (ed. G. Hunt). Arnold, London.
Montgomery, J. (1987) 'Confidentiality and the immature minor.' *Family Law*, **101**.
NHS Executive (1990) *Access to Health Records Act 1990: A Guide for the NHS*. NHSME, London.
Nightingale, F. (1859) *Notes on Nursing*. Blackie reprint 1974, Glasgow, pp. 70-71.
Royal College of Nurses (1991) *Guidelines on Confidentiality in Nursing*. RCN, London.
Scrivens, E. (1995) *Accreditation: Protecting the Professional or the Consumer*. Open University Press, Milton Keynes.
Seighart, P. (1982) 'Professional ethics: for whose benefit?' *Journal of Medical Ethics*, **8**.
Siegler, M. (1987) 'A decrepit concept.' *New England Journal of Medicine*, **307**, 1518.
Thompson, I. (1979) 'The nature of confidentiality.' *Journal of Medical Ethics*, **5**.
Turner, T. (1994) 'Paradox in practice.' *Nursing Times*, **90**(21), 18.
UKCC (1993) *Standards for Records and Record Keeping*. United Kingdom Central Council for Nursing, Midwifery and Health Visiting, London, (i) para 39; (ii) para 30.
UKCC (1996) *Guidelines for Professional Practice*. United Kingdom Central Council for Nursing, Midwifery and Health Visiting, London, (i) para 52; (ii) para 56; (iii) para 59; (iv) para 61; (v) para 64; (vi) para 40; (vii) para 41; (viii) para 64.
Working for Patients (1989) CM 555, London.

Chapter 8

Clinical research and the nurse

Jean McHale

Nurses increasingly participate in clinical trials. The nurse may run her or his own trial or may undertake research as part of a diploma qualification or for a higher degree. The nurse may be involved in a trial being run by a medical practitioner or by another nurse. A nurse may be a member of a research ethics committee which has the task of scrutinising proposals for clinical research in a particular area. This chapter provides an account of the legal regulation of research and the obligation of the researcher to the research subject. The basic principles on which research should be conducted are outlined in the document *Guidelines for Professional Practice* (UKCC, 1996(i)).

The first section considers the manner in which clinical research is regulated. In the second section, the role of research ethics committees in scrutinising clinical trials and legal principles regulating clinical trials are discussed. In the final section the question of negligence actions brought against nurses and others where research subjects are injured in a clinical trial are considered, along with the role of the nurse in policing unethical researchers.

Framework of regulation

The abuses of clinical research in Nazi Germany and in Japan during the middle years of this century resulted in pressure for the regulation of clinical research. International guidelines were developed, most notably the Nuremberg Code in 1949 and the Declaration of Helsinki in 1964. In this country there is no one piece of legislation governing the conduct of all research activity although certain legislation does govern specific areas such as animal research (Animals (Scientific Procedure) Act 1986) and research undertaken on embryos (Human Fertilisation and Embryology Act 1990). A number of guidelines have been published, for example by the Department of Health (DOH, 1991), the Royal College of Physicians

(RCP, 1996) and by the Royal College of Nursing (RCN, 1993). While these guidelines are not legally binding, they suggest conduct which amounts to good research practice and may be referred to in subsequent legal proceedings. The law governing research derives from general principles of civil law and criminal law, along with certain specific statutory provisions such as the Medicines Act 1968.

Clinical research is undertaken across a vast area of scientific activity. Certain research gives rise to particularly difficult ethical issues requiring careful consideration. Instances of this are the use of fetal tissue and the practice of gene therapy research. The latter is overseen by a specially created Government body, the Gene Therapy Advisory Committee, which imposes stringent requirements on researchers. This chapter focuses upon those clinical trials in which nurses are at present most likely to be involved, and discusses general principles of research activity on human subjects.

Drug trials and innnovative therapies

Before medicines are made available to the public they must be licensed by the Department of Health or the Department of Agriculture. Unlicensed medicines may be used if the Government has issued a clinical trial certificate. Such a certificate does not have to be obtained under what is known as the DDX provision if the trial is being conducted by a doctor, other than under arrangements with a manufacturer or supplier. If these requirements are not complied with then criminal penalties may follow (Dodds-Smith 1992). Although safeguards in the form of licensing exist in relation to experimental drug therapy, there are at present no equivalent safeguards as regards innovative therapy, such as keyhole surgery. Kennedy and Grubb (1994) have suggested that, in view of the fine line between innovative therapy and research, innovative therapy should be classed as medical research in situations in which the main purpose of therapy is to acquire knowledge, as opposed to care for the patient. In the light of much public concern regarding the use of certain new therapeutic techniques, notably keyhole surgery, the Government indicated that it was considering the introduction of legislation in this area (*The Times*, 21 February 1995). The Government has suggested that the Royal Medical Colleges should establish a committee on the safety and efficacy of medical intervention. New techniques would be referred to the committee. Small groups of experts would be given the task of deciding which techniques should be used and how their effectiveness should be assessed.

Animal research

The Animals Scientific Procedures Act 1986 states that before research can be undertaken on animals, researchers must obtain a licence from the Home Secretary. A Home Office committee examines whether the benefits to be gained from research being undertaken upon these animals justify the suffering which may be occasioned. The practice and ethics of these procedures go beyond the scope of the book and the reader is referred to further sources (see, for example, Fox, 1995).

Regulation of research

This section considers the basis of regulation of clinical research involving human subjects and legal principles governing the operation of clinical trials, as well as the criteria which the nurse should satisfy before embarking on a clinical trial. The principles of consent to treatment applicable in the context of research are considered, and the particular problems which arise in the context of certain groups of research subjects such as children and the mentally incompetent. A nurse researcher will also be bound to respect patient confidentiality, and particular applications of this are considered. This section concludes by examining the role and obligations of the nurse researcher on the wards.

Before a trial is undertaken, the researcher should obtain approval for the conduct of the trial from a research ethics committee. The main guidelines governing the operation of such committees are those issued by the Department of Health (DOH, 1991). These recommend that a local research ethics committee should be composed of between eight and 12 members drawn from hospital medical staff, nursing staff, general practitioners and two or more lay persons (DOH, 1991i). The guidelines suggest that the chair or the deputy chair should be a lay person. Lay members import a degree of independence into the decision-making process.

Where it is proposed to undertake a trial over a number of research centres in different health authority areas, the proposal should be referred to one of a number of newly created committees governing the approval of multicentred trials which have been established.

Assessing the risk

A researcher must satisfy the committee that the project is ethical and that any risk posed to research subjects is of an acceptable level. Factors which the committee must consider include any discomfort or distress the project may cause the research subject, any hazards which may arise during the project and precautions which should be introduced to deal with them, and the extent to which the research subject's health will be affected by involvement in a trial. The Royal College of Physicians (RCP, 1986) comments that 'a risk greater than minimal is not acceptable in a volunteer study'. However, what if a volunteer is prepared to accept that risk? Some people will take risks of a very high order for altruistic reasons. A person may volunteer to be involved in a trial to help researchers develop a cure for a condition suffered by a close relative. It is unclear whether it is lawful for a research subject to consent to involvement in a very high risk trial. As was noted earlier in relation to consent to treatment, English law does not allow a person to consent to any harm. If a research subject included in a high risk trial dies, then there is the possibility that a researcher would be prosecuted for manslaughter.

There has been controversy as to whether women of childbearing age should be included in a clinical trial and, in particular, concern as to the inclusion of women who are pregnant. That does not mean that trials cannot be undertaken on pregnant women. Indeed, trials into birthing techniques and the use of devices such as birth cushions require pregnant women of course! Those proposing to undertake such a trial should bear in mind the Department of Health (1991ii) guidelines which state:

> 'Where women are used as research subjects the possibility of their being or becoming pregnant should always be considered. The recruitment of females of child bearing age should always be justified by the researcher.'

Whether the possibility of risk to female volunteers of childbearing age from involvement in a clinical trial justifies their exclusion from such trials is the subject of much debate. While involvement may potentially harm such volunteers, it could be seen as paternalistic to ban involvement. Perhaps a better approach is to examine rigorously any trial where women of childbearing age are involved and to ensure that all women are provided with full information as to any possible risks to their health from involvement in the trial if they become pregnant.

Inducements to participate

Many trials are undertaken using volunteers. While some may be willing to give up their time out of altruism, many trials would simply not go ahead unless some inducements were given. A small financial inducement may be given to compensate for time spent and potential inconvenience caused. But while payment of small sums may be acceptable, there is a danger that an unethical researcher may offer large sums to encourage participation in a trial imposing an undue risk. Similarly, some payments to researchers may be unethical. If the researcher receives payment on the basis that the more patients are recruited the larger the fee, there is danger that researchers may place undue pressures on patients and others to be included in the research (DOH, 1991iii). Nonetheless, the level of any inducement given to the NHS body, health professionals, researchers or subjects to participate in clinical research is a factor that will be considered by a local research ethics committee when considering whether to approve a clinical trial (DOH, 1991iv). Inducements to research subjects may of course be other than financial. For example, pressure may be put on nurses by nurse researchers to participate in clinical trials because it is something which is expected of them. Such pressure is unjustifiable. It is important to ensure that subjects give full and free consent to entry into any trial.

Consent

As with any clinical procedure, it is vital to obtain consent from a research subject before a trial commences. The nurse may have the task of obtaining a patient's consent to participation in a trial or, even if not involved in initially obtaining consent, the nurse may be drawn into the process if a patient later approaches her or him and asks questions about the trial. Ensuring that research subjects are given adequate information is an important part of the role of a research ethics committee. What information must be given to the research subject in a clinical trial? A distinction should be drawn between therapeutic and non-therapeutic trials. Therapeutic research is research intended to benefit an individual patient. Non-therapeutic research is research which is unlikely to or will not benefit the research subject (whether a patient or healthy volunteer) personally.

The Department of Health guidelines provide simply that the research subject should give written consent and that the consent should be 'real'. While they state that a research subject should be given an information sheet before giving consent they do not specify the content of such an information sheet. The research ethics committee looks at the information sheet compiled by researchers to give to research subjects, to see if it is satisfactory. The Royal College of Physicians (1991i) recommends that information sheets should always contain statements regarding the nature of the investigation, the procedures involved, risks and possible benefits to the subject or others and the fact that a subject can decline to participate without giving reasons or incurring a penalty. In addition, if the research ethics committee decides that the risks warrant it, the Royal College recommends that the sheet should include statements as to the availability of compensation and also an invitation to research subjects to ask for further information. These are sensible recommendations. An information sheet should provide as full and clear an explanation as possible. But the nurse will not have fulfilled her or his legal obligations by simply handing over an information sheet. This issue is developed further below.

Providing full information recognises the autonomy of the research subject. Without informed consent, research subjects may not realise that they are being subjected to procedures aimed at benefiting future patients rather than themselves. However, there are certain situations in which researchers may wish to withhold information from patients. Take randomised controlled trials: some patients included in a trial recover not because of the effect of new medication, but simply because they think that they have been given a new drug. This is known as the 'placebo effect'. In an attempt to overcome this problem, researchers undertake randomised controlled trials. Research subjects are divided into two groups: one group is given the treatment, the other is given a placebo or dummy treatment. The patient does not know whether s/he is receiving the real or the dummy treatment. A variant on this is the 'double-blind' trial: in this type of trial, both the clinician and research subject do not know whether the patient has been given the treatment or an inert substance. It is particularly important for patients to appreciate that they are being entered into a randomised clinical trial and that there is a risk of missing out on a standard course of treatment. When providing information about the trial, researchers must ensure that all subjects are told that they are free to withdraw at any stage (DOH, 1991v).

There are no statutes or decided cases in English law stating how much information subjects in clinical trials should be given. A research subject may claim that provision of inadequate information constitutes the tort of battery. As stated earlier in relation to consent to medical treatment, the courts have stated that as long as a patient gives general consent to an operation being undertaken then health care professionals will not be liable in battery (*Chatterson* v. *Gerson* [1981] QB 432 at 443). But would the same test be applied to clinical research? In the Canadian case of *Halushka* v. *University of Satsatchewan* it was held that the failure of researchers to provide the subject with full information constituted a battery, Hall J.A. said:

> 'The subjects of medical experimentation are entitled to a full and frank disclosure of all the facts, probabilities and opinions which a reasonable man might be expected to consider before giving consent.([1965] 53 DLR (2d) 436 at 438).'

It is suggested that the adoption of such an approach, requiring a broad duty of disclosure to those entering a non-therapeutic trial, is desirable. What of patients included in therapeutic trials? The difficulty here is that if patients included in trials had to be given full explanation this would give such patients the right to receive more information than a patient receiving any other therapy. At present it seems likely that the courts would hold that a patient is entitled to the same level of disclosure whether therapy is given as part of treatment or as therapeutic research.

It may be necessary to undertake research using patients brought in unconscious into casualty and who are in a critical condition. The Department of Health (1991vi) guidelines provide that the research projects involving such patients should be examined with particular care. If it is possible to anticipate that a patient may be subject to an unexpected event, such as complications during childbirth, then the researchers should obtain the patient's consent before labour begins.

Duty to inform - negligence

While a research subject may have been given some information as to the trial such that an action in battery may be difficult to establish, a research subject may claim that a researcher acted negligently because inadequate information was provided as to the risks posed by involvement in the trial. In the context of medical treatment, as discussed earlier a nurse is not negligent as long as s/he gives the patient such information as would have been provided by a responsible body of professional nursing opinion (*Sidaway* v. *Bethlem Royal Hospital Governors* [1985] AC 871). Does the duty differ in relation to clinical research?

Two alternative approaches could be taken. Given the uncertain nature of clinical research and the risks involved, a different standard of disclosure could be adopted for treatment and therapeutic research. The research subject could be entitled to receive more information than the patient. But the dividing line between therapeutic treatment and therapeutic research is a very fine one and this may be regarded as an unjustifiably narrow distinction to draw. Alternatively, a complete reassessment could be made of the legal obligation to disclose information to patients. It appears unlikely that the courts or Parliament will attempt such a reform in the near future. Such judicial or legislative reform may not prove necessary if clinical practice moves towards providing patients routinely with information regarding the risks of treatment (see Chapter 5).

A strong argument can be made in favour of full disclosure of all risks in the case of non-therapeutic trials. If a research subject is subjected to scientific tests for the benefit of the community as a whole and not for his or her own personal benefit then s/he should be told of the risks run by involvement in the project.

What must be emphasised is that to simply provide a large amount of information about potential risks of entry into a clinical trial may be of little value. A nurse will not comply with his or her legal obligation by simply providing a patient with an information sheet. The RCN (1993) suggests that the researcher should:

> 'explain as fully as possible, and in terms meaningful to the subjects, the nature and the purpose of the study, how and why they were selected and invited to take part, what is required of them and who is undertaking and financing the investigation.'

The nurse can independently observe what information the patient has been given. S/he may be of the view that the information which has been given is inadequate. In such a situation, the nurse should raise the concerns with the researcher. It is certainly arguable that in a research situation the nurse may be justified in personally providing the research subject with more information. However, the nurse should only contemplate providing the patient with more information directly after having ascertained the position regarding disclosure. The question of unethical researchers is explored further in the section on policing trials below. See also discussion of conflicts between nurses and other health care professionals over information disclosure on page 76.

Where a research subject asks questions about the research project, again whether the researcher has to fully answer such queries is unclear. It is submitted that, as with medical treatment, any refusal to provide information would require careful justification in the case of a therapeutic trial, and that such a refusal would be unjustifiable in the case of a non-therapeutic trial.

Can patients be compelled to participate?

Consider a patient asked to participate in a clinical trial. The trial offers the prospect of a cure for what is otherwise an incurable condition. The patient refuses to be involved. Could the patient be compelled to participate? The law states that a competent adult patient has the right to refuse treatment, even if as a consequence the patient dies. In a number of controversial cases (see Chapter 6) in which treatment has been authorised despite patient refusal. Nonetheless, it is doubtful whether any court would authorise the inclusion of a competent but protesting adult in a research trial, even if the trial was clearly therapeutic. Indeed to sanction such involvement would, it is submitted, represent an unjustifiable limitation on individual autonomy.

If a nurse or doctor in charge of a project appears to be putting pressure on a patient to participate, the nurse acting as patient advocate, should make the patient aware of his or her right to refuse to be included in the trial. The nurse should also protest to the researcher about what s/he regards as bad practice. If a researcher continues to act in flagrant disregard of legal obligations, then the nurse should bring the matter to the attention of the appropriate bodies, including the research ethics committee.

Children and clinical trials

Wherever possible, clinical trials should be conducted using competent adults (DOH, 1991vii). But in some situations it is necessary to include children in a clinical trial, for instance if the trial involves a study into childhood diseases, or the suitability for administration to children of a drug which is currently used to treat adult patients. A research ethics committee assesses the risk level of trials. The risk to a child of participation in a trial is something which the research ethics committee will be particularly concerned to assess.

Particular difficulties surround non-therapeutic trials. The Department of Health (1991viii) guidelines emphasise that to expose a child in a non-therapeutic trial to a risk other than merely negligible may be to act unlawfully. But is this right? We noted earlier that some are of the view that it is legitimate to include children in non-therapeutic procedures as long as this is 'not against' their best interests. It has been argued that just as parents are lawfully entitled to expose their children to certain quite risky activities they should be entitled to expose them to the risks surrounding entry into a clinical trial (Nicholson, 1985). One approach is to limit the entry of child patients to those trials where there is minimal risk, an approach for example favoured by the British Paediatric Association (BPA, 1992). But there is scope for disagreement as to what constitutes 'minimal risk'. A scientist may rate a procedure as having a lower risk than would a patient assessing the same procedure (Nicholson, 1991). Research ethics committees need to be extremely sensitive to the different weightings which may be placed on risk levels by scientists and research subjects in scrutinising research protocols.

If it is proposed to include a child in a clinical trial, from whom should patient consent be obtained - parent or child? As already discussed, in law, a child over 16 years can give consent to medical treatment and a child under that age may be competent to give consent (s8 Family Law Reform Act 1969). In *Gillick* v. *West Norfolk and Wisbech AHA* ([1985] 3 All ER 402), the House of Lords held that whether a child under 16 years was capable of consenting to medical treatment was dependent upon an assessment of the child's maturity. It seems likely that the *Gillick* approach would be adopted by a court if it was asked to consider whether a child could consent to involvement in a therapeutic research project. Application of this test is not straightforward. Researchers must assess carefully each child individually to determine his or her capacity to consent to be involved in a particular trial. It would be good practice for researchers to ensure that they have the written consent of those with parental responsibility, even if the child is competent to consent to involvement in the trial.

It is uncertain whether a child can consent to being included in a non-therapeutic trial. The courts may be prepared to adopt the *Gillick* test of competency and hold that a competent child may give a valid consent to involvement in a non-therapeutic research project. But would a child be competent to make that choice? It is important not to underestimate a child's powers of comprehension. Mason and McCall Smith (1994) comment that it would be very unusual for a child in his or her teens not to understand the implications of entry into a clinical trial.

Compelling a child to be involved

What can a nurse do if a child tearfully refuses to be involved in the project? Can the child be compelled on the grounds that it is in his or her best interests to be involved? The courts have indicated that if a competent child refuses treatment, the parents may authorise treatment on the child's behalf. Compelling a child's involvement in any clinical procedure is a very serious step. Were such conflicts to arise and the issue go to court, then it is submitted that a court is unlikely to authorise a child to be forcibly involved in a therapeutic trial, save perhaps in an exceptional situation where the child is suffering from a condition with a terminal prognosis and the treatment represents the child's only chance of life. Even here, it would be exceedingly controversial to compel involvement.

Can a very young child be forced to take part in a clinical trial? The Department of Health guidelines do not deal with this question. The legal position is uncertain. Certainly, as far as possible, the wishes of even a very young child should be given serious consideration in making this decision (also refer to page 83).

The incompetent adult

The nurse may be involved in a research project including mentally ill or mentally handicapped adults. Wherever possible, competent adult subjects should be used. But, as with the child subject, there may be situations in which research is inevitable on the mentally ill and incompetent because it relates to a condition specific to this subject group, such as, for example, research into a particular mental illness or the effects of a particular treatment. For example, a study into the side effects of antipsychotic drugs must be undertaken using clients who are receiving such medication. However, researchers must not forget that while persons may have some mental impairment, this does not mean that they are totally unable to give consent. The majority of psychiatric patients are as capable of giving consent as other patients (Royal College of Psychiatrists, 1990). Admittedly, some patients will never reach that level of competence. Nevertheless, including such patients in a research project may be of very real benefit to them or to groups of other patients in the future.

As stated in Chapter 6, relatives and other persons have no power to give consent in law on behalf of a mentally incompetent person. The House of Lords in *Re F* ([1990] 2 AC 1) stated that treatment may be given where the health professionals believe that it is in the best interests of an incompetent patient. While the question of therapeutic research was not discussed in *Re F*, it appears likely that such research may be justified if it can be shown that it is treatment for 'life, health, well-being'. The difficulty lies in determining what amounts to treatment in the 'best interests' of the patient. In *Re F*, Lord Brandon said:

> 'The operation or other treatment will be in the best interests of such patients if, but only if, it is carried out either in order to save their lives or in order to ensure improvement/prevent deterioration in their physical/mental health.'

As far as non-therapeutic research is concerned, at present it appears that it is unlawful to undertake non-therapeutic research on a mentally incompetent patient. It can be argued that such research is not in the best interests of a mentally incompetent adult within the definition of the House of Lords in *Re F*.

Concern as to the vulnerability of the mentally incompetent adult, and the need to ensure that procedures were undertaken only when necessary, is reflected in the report of the Law Commission on Mental Incapacity (HMSO, 1995). It accepted that in certain limited situations non-therapeutic research could be undertaken, but subject to safeguards. First, all non-therapeutic trials on mentally incompetent adults should be referred to a specially created committee, a mental incapacity research committee. Such a committee would examine whether intended research projects satisfied a number of criteria:

'1. that it is desirable to provide knowledge of the causes or treatment of, or of the care of people affected by, the incapacitating condition with which any participant is affected;
2. that the object of the research cannot be effectively achieved without the participation of persons who are or who may be without capacity to consent, and
3. that the research will not expose a participant to more than a negligible risk, will not be unduly invasive or restrictive of a participant and will not unduly interfere with a participant's freedom of action or privacy. (Draft Bill clause 11(3))'

The committee was to approve trial proposals in principle. Involvement of a particular individual in a trial was a matter to be assessed separately. First, some of the participants may give consent themselves. The Law Commission gave the example of proposed research upon members of a residential home who have Alzheimer's disease. If individuals are unable to themselves give consent, the Law Commission recommended that research may be undertaken where there has been court approval, consent of an attorney or manager, certificate from a doctor not involved in the research that the person's participation is appropriate or that the research is designated as one which does not involve direct contact (draft Bill clause 11(1)(c) and (4)). This final consideration refers to covert observation, photography or the inspection of written records. Allowing automatic approval for such observational studies is exceedingly controversial. Much may depend upon the condition of the individual patient. Any decision to include a person in such a project should be made on the basis of what constitutes that person's best interests.

Confidentiality and research information

Nurses must always bear in mind that patient information is to be treated as confidential. Research projects may involve highly sensitive clinical information, for example a study examining counselling provision for persons who are HIV positive. The nurse, as we saw earlier, is obliged by his or her contract of employment and by the UKCC professional ethical code to maintain patient confidentiality. The RCN (1993) has stated that:

> 'usually this means that data are analysed and reported in such a way that particular individuals, small groups or even organisations cannot be identified unless they have given prior agreement, the full information being only known to the research team.'

Research may be undertaken using existing medical records. In principle, the patient's consent to disclosure should be obtained. However, if the sample is very large, tracing all patients may be totally impracticable. Nevertheless, the Department of Health guidelines stress that if a patient has previously indicated that s/he did not want his or her medical information released for the purposes of medical research, this request should be respected (DOH, 1991).

It is important that information generated during a clinical trial is kept just as confidential as any other clinical information. The researcher must respect the confidentiality of information given to him or her by staff and patients. Unauthorised disclosure is not only ethically unjustifiable, but it may also prejudice further research. If a study is undertaken into working practices on the wards, it is important to ensure that nurses can speak frankly. They may not be willing to be so frank without a guarantee of anonymity being provided and adhered to. No individual should be identifiable from the published results without consent. The Department of Health guidelines emphasise that identifiable data should be destroyed at the end of the project if no longer needed by the researcher (DOH, 1991). If the researcher wants to keep the data, he or she must be prepared to justify this to the research ethics committee/relevant NHS body and to the research subject.

The Department of Health recommends that persons should not be included in the trial unless they agree that information can be disclosed to their GP. On the face of it, this may seem a perfectly reasonable suggestion. Without that information, a GP subsequently treating the patient may not realise that certain symptoms are related to involvement in a clinical trial. But that does not mean that it is desirable for all information to be automatically transferred. What if, for example, tests are undertaken and it is found that the research subject has tested HIV positive? The subject may be unwilling for this information to be passed on to the GP. The author suggests that any rule requiring disclosure to a GP should not be absolute in nature.

Intervention with care of the patient on the ward

While observing practice on the ward, the nurse researcher may come across situations in which patient care falls below what is regarded as being an acceptable standard (Dines, 1995):

> 'A nurse researcher is interested in the feeding problems of stroke patients. She is using non-participant observation as her research method. She is seated inconspicuously wearing a white coat in the ward; it is a meal time. A stroke patient nearby is propped up against his pillows and reaches for his milky tea. He takes the spouted beaker to his lips but spills the drink down his pyjama jacket. No nurse is in sight, what should the nurse researcher do?'

'Some time later the sister appears; she is updating the fluid balance charts. Observing the empty beaker she congratulates the patient on drinking his tea and charts the fluid intake. What should the nurse researcher do?'

Should the nurse intervene? As Dines notes, the nurse faces a dilemma. By intervening she would be unable to observe what action the ward sister would take in that situation, a matter which is part of her research. But if the nurse failed to act and the patient became dehydrated would she be negligent? In this situation a court would have to consider whether she owed a duty to the patient on that ward. The nurse is not responsible directly for the clinical care of that patient. There is no general duty to act as a 'Good Samaritan'. If the nurse researcher was held to be under a duty in such a situation, the court would assess whether the conduct was negligent by reference to a responsible body of professional practice. Some guidance to the approach of one body of professional opinion in such a situation can be gleaned from a publication of the RCN. The RCN (1993) suggests that:

'The nurse who is undertaking a research project in an exclusively research role has no responsibility for the service, care, treatment or advice given to patients or clients unless stipulated within the design of the research. Otherwise, any intervention in a professional capacity should be confined to situations in which a patient or client requires to be protected or rescued from danger.'

But it is uncertain what is meant here by 'protection from danger'. Does this mean immediate danger or something which becomes dangerous because it is repeated - the patient regularly spilling his or her drink and losing fluid?
The RCN (1993) has said:

'A nurse in a research situation still holds expert knowledge and may at times feel impelled to action for a patient's benefit.'

Whether the nurse is held to be negligent may depend on factors such as the risk to the patient by her non-intervention. Take the example given at the start of this section. If the nurse continued to observe the patient losing fluids and that no check was made by the sister and the patient was placed at grave risk of dehydration, then it is arguable that by not acting to warn the nurse on the ward the nurse researcher would be negligent.

Compensating research subjects and policing trials

This section considers liability of nurses, whether as researchers or as ethics committee members when trials go wrong. Also discussed is the role of the nurse in policing unethical behaviour in a trial. As noted above, the general principles of law apply to clinical trials. If a research subject is not told of a particular risk of involvement in a trial and that risk materialises and the subject is injured s/he may bring an action in negligence or battery against the researcher. If a research subject is injured during a trial due to the researcher's lack of care, then again an action for negligence may be brought.

No national scheme of compensation exists for those injured in clinical trials. Researchers must be adequately insured. However, some special compensation provision exists for certain trials. The Association of British Pharmaceutical Industries (ABPI) guidelines provide that researchers should make contractually binding undertakings with research subjects in non-therapeutic trials to pay compensation in the event of injury. The Association does not require contractually binding undertakings to be made with research subjects, although it suggests that assurances should be given that compensation would be paid in the event of harm resulting. While there are no contractual sanctions for breaking an undertaking, to break it would lead to criticism and would make it very difficult for the researcher to arrange insurance cover from the Association in the future. This scheme has not, however, met with universal approval.

There has been some criticism of the operation of indemnity schemes by the ABPI in that it has installed threshold limits before claims can be brought (Burris, 1995). If the research is commissioned by the Medical Research Council there is no automatic entitlement to compensation, although the Council has indicated that compensation payments may be made on an *ex gratia* basis.

Liability of ethics committee members

If a research subject is injured in a clinical trial then it is possible that an action could be brought against individual members of the research ethics committee on the grounds that they were negligent in approving the conduct of the trial. It has been suggested that, at least in theory, each individual ethics committee member owes a duty of care to each research subject (Brazier, 1990). Any costs of legal proceedings brought against a nurse employed by the NHS who sits on a research ethics committee will be covered by NHS indemnity insurance. The Department of Health has stated that it will cover the costs of a research ethics committee member as long as s/he has not been guilty of misconduct or gross lack of care. It should be noted that although an action in negligence is a theoretical possibility, in practice bringing such a claim may be difficult. A research subject would have to show that it was the negligence of a particular committee member in approving the trial which caused the injury which s/he had suffered.

What can be done if it is thought that the trial is being conducted unethically?

If the nurse believes that a trial in which s/he is involved is being conducted unethically, the nurse may raise this with the person in charge of the trial. But what if no notice is taken of what the nurse has said? S/he can draw the matter to the attention of the research ethics committee who approved the trial. The committee may decide to take action, but in practice it has few powers. It may ask the researchers to report to them and then withdraw authorisation from the trial. If the unethical researcher is a nurse, it may be thought appropriate to refer the researcher's conduct to the UKCC, who may decide to take disciplinary proceedings. In the case of a doctor, misconduct may be referred to the General Medical Council.

If a nurse conducting a trial departs from an agreed trial protocol and has acted unethically it may limit the nurse's chances of obtaining approval for another clinical trial. But there is no national code stating how research ethics committees should scrutinise projects once these are up and running. While some committees have follow up procedures and write to the researcher to find out how the project has progressed, others do not. It is arguable that the rights of the subject in the trial are being neglected. Neuberger (1992) has suggested that new powers be given to committees to carry out spot checks. In addition, perhaps questionnaires could be given to research subjects to discover how a trial has been conducted. But to expect the research ethics committee to undertake detailed policing of the many trials which they scrutinise is unrealistic. Committee members are unpaid. Systematic scrutiny with spot checks, etc. would really require full time officers to be appointed. The administrative workload would increase, as would the cost. In an NHS subject to considerable budgetary restraints, such innovations are unlikely, at least in the immediate future.

References

Arras, J.D. (1990) 'Non-compliance in AIDS research.' *Hastings Center Report* , **20**, 24.

Brazier, M. (1990) 'The liability of ethics committee members.' *Professional Negligence*, **6**, 186.

British Paediatric Association (1992) *Guidelines for the Ethical Conduct of Research Involving Children*. BPA, London.

Burris, J.M. (1995) 'The compensation of patients injured in clinical trials.' *Journal of Medical Ethics*, **21**, 166.

Department of Health (1991) *Guidelines for Local Research Ethics Committees*. DOH, London, (i) para 2.5; (ii) para 4.5; (iii) para 7.86; (iv) para 3.15; (v) para 3.7; (vi) para 3.9; (vii) para 4.1; (viii) para 4.4.

Dines, A. (1995) 'An ethical perspective – nursing research.' In *Nursing Law and Ethics* (eds J. Tingle and A. Cribb). Blackwell Scientific, Oxford.

Dodds-Smith, I. (1992) 'Clinical research.' In *Doctors, Patients and the Law* (ed. C. Dyer). Blackwell Scientific, Oxford.

Fox, M. (1995) 'Animal rights and wrongs: medical ethics and the killing of non-human animals.' In *Death Rites: Law and Ethics at the End of Life* (eds R. Lee and D. Morgan). Routledge, London.

Kennedy, I. and Grubb, A. (1994) *Medical Law Text with Materials*, 2nd edn. Butterworths, London.

Kirk, E. (1995) 'Research and patients.' In *Nursing Law and Ethics* (eds J. Tingle and A. Cribb). Blackwell Scientific, Oxford.

Law Commission (1995) *Mental Incapacity*. Report No. 231, HMSO, London.

Mason, J.K. and McCall Smith, R.A. (1994) *Law and Medical Ethics*, 4th edn. Butterworths, London, p. 372.

Neuberger, J. (1992) *Ethics and Health Care; The Role of the Research Ethics Committee*. Kings Fund Institute, London.

Nicholson R. (1991) 'The ethics of research with children.' In *Protecting the Vulnerable* (eds M. Brazier and M. Lobjoit). Routledge, London.

Nicholson R. (1985) *Medical Research and Children*, MRC, London.

Royal College of Nursing (1993) *Ethics Relating to Research in Nursing*. Scutari Press, Harrow, (i) para 3.14.

Royal College of Physicians (1991) *Report of Working Party on Research on Patients* (i) para 7.12.

Royal College of Physicians (1986) *Research on Healthy Volunteers*, RCP, London.

Royal Colege of Physicians (1996) *Guidelines on the Practice of Ethics Committees in Medical Research Involving Human Subjects.* RCP, London.

Royal College of Psychiatrists (1990) 'Guidelines for Psychiatric research involving Human subjects.' *Psychiatric Bulletin*, **48**.

Royal Commission on Civil Liability for Personal Injury. 'Medical injury,' Chapter 24, para 1341.

Silverman, W.A. (1989) 'The myth of informed consent.' *Journal of Medical Ethics*, 251.

UKCC (1996) *Guidelines for Professional Practice*. United Kingdom Central Council for Nursing, Midwifery and Health Visiting, London, (i) para 82-87(ii).

Chapter 9

The nurse and the employment relationship

Jean McHale

As stated in Chapter 1, the nurse as a professional is subject to regulation by law and registered nurses are also subject to regulation by their professional organisation, the United Kingdom Central Council for Nursing, Midwifery and Health Visiting (UKCC). The nurse is also an employee and thus subject to the obligations imposed upon her or him by an employer, and should s/he breach the obligation they may also be disciplined by the employer. Breach of certain ethical requirements, for example breach of confidentiality, may render the nurse liable in law, before the UKCC and in addition before her or his employer (see Chapter 7). This chapter focuses upon the nurse's position as employee and considers some of the rights and obligations of that position. An overview of this area is provided; for more detailed discussion readers are referred to specialist texts (Smith and Thomas, 1996; Deakin and Morris, 1995).

The first section considers questions of recruitment and the legal nature of the employment relationship. The next section explores the obligations placed on both employer and employee to ensure a safe working environment, and presents a general overview of health and safety legislation. The third section considers particular problems regarding situations in which nurses may pose a risk to patients through, for example, illness. The final section examines the position of the nurse who suffers injury in the workplace and what redress is available to her.

The nurse and the employer

Contract of employment

When the nurse accepts the offer of a post, whether with a NHS trust or a private employer, s/he will enter into a contract of employment. The terms of the contract of employment may be written or oral. In the past, NHS employment contracts have been agreed nationally and fixed in relation to Whitley Council agreements. However, in the future the situation will change as NHS trusts negotiate terms on a local basis. Where a hospital becomes an NHS trust, employment contracts are transferred to the trust (s6 National Health Service and Community Care Act 1990). In such a situation the nurse's contract of employment cannot be altered without the nurse having been consulted.

As employees nurses have a statutory right to a written statement of certain information concerning their employment (s1 Employment Rights Act 1996). Information which may be requested includes the scale of pay, terms and conditions of service, job title and description. This applies to those employed for more than a month and who work for more than 8 hours a week (s198 Employment Rights Act 1996). The employee is also entitled to an itemised pay statement (s8 Employment Rights Act 1996).

Rights to paid and unpaid leave

In certain circumstances the nurse has the right to claim paid or unpaid leave. For example, if a nurse becomes a justice of the peace or a member of a local authority s/he may claim reasonable unpaid time off (s50(1) Employment Rights Act 1996). Nurses who undertake the functions of a trade union official also have a statutory right to paid leave (s168 Trade Union and Labour Relations Act 1992). Those employees who are not trade union officials also have a right to reasonable time off work to participate in trade union activities (s170 Trade Union and Labour Relations Act 1992).

Employees who are pregnant may claim paid leave under statutory maternity rights (s164 Social Security Contributions and Benefits Act 1992). In addition rights exist to statutory sick pay for a period of 14 weeks (also see below Rights of the Pregnant Employee).

Rights of the pregnant employee

The law contains special provisions regarding pregnant employees. First, to dismiss a woman on the grounds that she is pregnant will form the basis for an action for unfair dismissal (s99 Employment Rights Act 1996). Provisions of European law have been interpreted to the effect that to subject a woman to less favourable treatment because she is pregnant may constitute discrimination on the basis of sex and is unlawful (EC Directive 76/207 *Webb* v. *EMO Air Cargo (UK)* [1994] IRCR 482 EC2).

Statute accords pregnant women specific rights during and after the maternity period. Employees may claim paid leave for antenatal appointments (s55 Employment Rights Act 1996). After the first appointment the employer may require the woman to show a certificate from the doctor/midwife that she is pregnant, and her appointment card (s55 (2) (3) Employment Rights Act 1996). Pregnant women are entitled to a period of maternity leave; there is an entitlement to 14 weeks standard leave of absence (s71 Employment Rights Act 1996). She must give 21 days notice to her employer as to the fact that she is pregnant, the period of confinement and her intention to exercise her right to maternity leave. She must also notify the employer of her intention to return to work (s80, 82 1996 Act). This notice must be given at least 21 days before she proposes to return (s82, 1996 Act).

It should be noted that many NHS trusts provide more generous arrangements than are required under statute. In some instances employees are allowed to defer return for up to 5 years provided specified criteria are fulfilled for maintaining professional skills, and subject to the availability of a suitable post (Du Fen and Warwick, 1995). If a nurse returns to work after maternity leave she is entitled to return to a post at the same level as that which she left (s79 Employment Rights Act 1996).

A trust may decide to suspend a nurse in a situation in which her job poses a threat to her health and safety during pregnancy, has recently given birth or is breastfeeding the child (s66 Employment Rights Act 1996). The trust is under an obligation to see if there is suitable alternative employment which can be offered (s66–s67 Employment Rights Act 1996). If the nurse is suspended, then s/he is entitled to be paid at the level at which s/he was being paid before the suspension occurred, unless it is the case that the nurse has unreasonably refused substitute work (s68 Employment Rights Act 1996).

Discrimination on the basis of race, sex or disability

A nurse, as is the case in relation to any other employee, is entitled to respect and equal treatment regardless of race, sex or disability. The Race Relations Act 1976 and Sex Discrimination Act 1975 provide protection to both job applicants and to employees in post (s6(1), s33 Sex Discrimination Act 1975). The legislation covers both direct and indirect discrimination.

'Direct discrimination' refers to one person being treated less favourably than another on basis of their race or sex (s1(1)(a) Sex Discrimination Act 1975; s1(1) Race Relations Act 1976). 'Indirect discrimination' refers to a condition applied to an employee such that the proportion of persons of one race or sex who can comply with it is considerably smaller than the proportion of another, and where an employer cannot show that the condition is justifiable, and that it is to the detriment of the person to whom it applies (s1(1)(b) Sex Discrimination Act 1975; Race Relations Act 1976). If, for example, the job is one in which one sex requires privacy, such as toilet attendants, then discrimination may be justifiable.

Discrimination under the Sex Discrimination Act 1975 also extends to sexual harassment (*Porcelli* v. *Strathclyde Regional Council* [1986] ICR 564). Persons who are victimised because they take proceedings under the discrimination legislation (whether sex, race discrimination or the Equal

Pay Act 1970) are also afforded statutory protection (s4 Sex Discrimination Act 1975; s2 Race Relations Act 1976). Initially, male midwives were a recognised exception to the general law on discrimination, but this was altered in 1983. Nevertheless, regulations allow women to choose to be attended by a female midwife. Where a male midwife does attend a women in childbirth, arrangements should be made to ensure that he is accompanied (1983 SI No. 1202). If a person is treated less favourably because s/he has complained about discrimination, then this may constitute 'victimisation' and an employee may also seek redress under the legislation.

The Equal Pay Act 1970 (as amended) also allows claims to be brought by persons in existing employment relationships who believe that they are being discriminated against in their terms and conditions of employment. This has to be seen today in the light of developments in the European Union such as Article 119 of the Treaty of Rome, which provides that member states shall 'ensure and subsequently maintain the principle that men and women shall receive equal pay for equal work'. Further consideration of this legislation goes beyond the scope of this book (see Smith and Thomas, 1996i).

Legislation recently extended protection against discrimination to persons with a disability. The Disability Discrimination Act 1995 provides that it is unlawful for an employer to discriminate against a disabled person in offering employment and, once employed, in relation to their terms and conditions of employment (s1(1) Disability Discrimination Act 1995). Disability as defined in the Act refers to individuals who have a

> 'physical or mental impairment which has a substantial or long term adverse effect on their ability to carry out normal day to day activities.'

It appears that impairment for the purposes of this legislation is not intended to include addictions or anti-social behaviour.

An employer discriminates against a disabled person if, for a reason related to their disability, the employer treats them less fairly than he would treat others who do not have a disability (s5 Disability Discrimination Act 1995). An employer can only discriminate if s/he can show that this discrimination was justifiable. Situations in which discrimination is justifiable are set out in section 5. For example, it can be justifiable to discriminate if a person's disability is such as to significantly impede performance of that person's duties. Complaints regarding discrimination should be brought before an industrial tribunal within a period of 3 months of the action being complained of (s8(1) and schedule 3 para 1). In addition to the 1995 Act the Disabled Persons Employment Act 1994 imposes a quota on all employers to employ disabled persons where the organisation employs more than 20 persons. The standard quota is 3%.

The Race Relations Act 1976 and Sex Discrimination Act 1975 are monitored by the Commission for Racial Equality and the Equal

Opportunities Commission. These bodies have both supervisory and enforcement roles. Matters may be referred to them to undertake investigations. If they find that discrimination has taken place, they may issue enforcement proceedings. In some situations they may issue legal proceedings where discriminatory conduct has taken place. For example, they have particular powers to take legal action where discriminatory advertisements have been published (s38 Sex Discrimination Act 1975). They also publish documents regarding good practice. Practice in the NHS has from time to time been subject to investigation regarding claims of discrimination, for example, under-representation of ethnic minorities in lower nursing grades.

An individual who has suffered discrimination may bring an action before an industrial tribunal or, in the case of sex and race discrimination, may take the case to the Equal Opportunities Commission or the Commission for Racial Equality, which may decide to bring proceedings.

Trade union rights

A nurse may join a trade union. Equally, the nurse has the right to resign and not be unjustifiably expelled from the trade union (Part III Trade Union and Labour Relations (Consolidation) Act 1992). A trade union may set out requirements for membership, but otherwise it must admit anyone who seeks to join the organisation. Union rules cannot deny an individual employee access to the courts of law. Legislation also requires that the employee may not be unjustifiably disciplined by a union (s64 Trade Union and Labour Relations (Consolidation) Act 1992). For further consideration of this complex topic readers are referred to specialist texts on the subject and advised to seek specialist legal advice (Smith and Thomas, 1996ii; Morris and Archer, 1993).

Dismissal

An employee who believes that s/he has been unjustifiably dismissed may bring an action on the basis that the dismissal was 'wrongful' or 'unfair'. This may be because s/he has been dismissed or because while the nurse has resigned the circumstances under which the resignation took place amount to what is known as 'constructive dismissal' on the part of the employer. A claim for wrongful dismissal may be brought to the common law courts. However, the remedy is limited to, in effect, loss of earnings for the applicable notice period. In practice, it is more likely that an employee will bring a claim of unfair dismissal before an industrial tribunal.

Unfair dismissal

An employee who believes that s/he was unjustifiably dismissed may bring an action claiming unfair dismissal before an industrial tribunal (s94 and s98–s99 Employment Rights Act 1996). An instance of such a case was discussed in Chapter 7 in relation to the nurse Graham Pink who alleged that one reason for his dismissal concerned the fact that he had blown the whistle on what he saw as misconduct (see section *Conflicts between confidentiality and the need to uphold standards of care*). Where a hearing takes place, a tribunal determines whether the dismissal was unfair by asking was the employer's conduct 'reasonable' in accordance with equity and the substantial merits of the case. Unfairness may be as to the substance of the decision or as to the procedures used. The decision must fall within the 'band of reasonableness'. If the employee's claim is upheld then s/he may be reinstated to her or his job, or may receive compensation. In practice, compensation is the likely remedy, because in only a very tiny proportion of cases will an employee be reinstated to the original job.

Safety and the workplace

Both nurse and employer are under legal obligations in relation to workplace safety. Health and safety at work is the subject of detailed legislative provisions and also regulation through European directives. This section highlights some ways in which the nurse may be affected by health and safety legislation.

The Health and Safety at Work etc. Act 1974 and subsequent legislation places duties upon both employers and employees. Initially, this legislation did not apply to NHS bodies because they were covered by what was known as 'Crown immunity'. This immunity was removed in 1990 (s60 National Health Service and Community Care Act 1990).

Health and safety in the workplace is supervised by a number of organisations which have been established under the Health and Safety at Work etc. Act 1974. The Health and Safety Commission (HSC) (schedule 2 para 15) oversees the work of the Health and Safety Executive (HSE). It establishes policy in relation to health and safety risks, and produces and keeps under review guidance in the forms of codes of practice. The Commission lays down policy guidelines for inspectorates, makes proposals for new legislation and encourages research.

Another body, the Health and Safety Executive, has the task of actually enforcing the legislation (s18(1) Health and Safety at Work Act 1974). Health and Safety Executive inspectors have wide ranging powers to enter premises, ask questions, take samples, make measurements, take photographs and scrutinise or seize documents (s20 Health and Safety at Work Act 1974). Inspectors visit places of work. Visits may take place because inspectors have been notified that an accident has taken place, or they have received a complaint. If an inspector finds that a piece of legislation has been infringed s/he may issue an improvement notice stating what is wrong and requiring it to be remedied (1974 Act s21). Alternatively, if something is being done which in the inspector's opinion carries the risk of serious injury, then s/he may issue a prohibition notice ordering that the activity be stopped either immediately or on a specified future date (1974 Act s22). An appeal may be made against these notices to an industrial tribunal. Ultimately, if the notice is not complied with, the Health and Safety inspector may prosecute the employer in the magistrates' court.

Within the Health and Safety Executive is a special body known as the Employment Medical Advisory Service (EMAS). EMAS is staffed primarily by qualified occupational nurses and physicians. EMAS provides advice to employers, employees and bodies such as trade unions on the effect of employment on health. Members of EMAS have powers to undertake regular examination of persons employed in known hazardous occupations. The employer is required to provide his or her employee with details of this service (Management of Health and Safety Executive SI 1992 No 205 1989).

The 1974 Act provides that an employer, whether trust or GP, shall do all that is reasonably practicable to ensure the health, safety and welfare of its employees and that they are not exposed to undue risks (s2 and s3 Health and Safety at Work Act 1974). Failure to comply with these provisions is a criminal offence. The law requires employees to be given such information, instruction, training and supervision as is necessary to ensure their health and safety, including information as to any special health risks which they may run (Management of Health and Safety at Work Regulations SI 1992 No 205 1992).

The obligations regarding health and safety are imposed upon employees as well as employers. Section 7 of the Health and Safety at Work Act 1974 provides that employees must:

> 'take reasonable care for the health and safety of other persons who may be affected by his acts or omissions at work and
>
> as regards any duty or requirement imposed on his employer or any other person by relevant statutory provisions to cooperate with him so far as is necessary to enable that duty or requirement to be performed or complied with.'

Breach of this duty is a criminal offence and punishment on conviction is usually a fine. Even if the decision is taken not to prosecute a nurse for breach of section 7, the nurse is still at risk of dismissal for failing to comply with health and safety arrangements. Failure to comply with training requirements in health and safety also places the nurse at risk of prosecution or dismissal. Where accidents take place at work a report must be compiled and the relevant authorities notified.

One way in which safe practices in the workplace may be monitored is through the safety representative and the safety committee. Legislation provides for the appointment of safety representatives by trade unions - a nurse may be appointed on to a safety committee at her or his hospital by the nurse's trade union (section 2(4) Health and Safety at Work Act

1974). The safety representative has the task of investigating potential hazards and dangerous occurrences. S/he has statutory rights to inspect the workplace on a routine basis. Employers must also consult safety representatives on a number of matters such as the introduction of changes in workplace health and safety and the provision of information (Management of Health and Safety at Work Regulations SI 1992 No. 2051). Employers may also establish safety committees, and indeed in some situations are required to do so. A safety committee is a small committee with equivalent employee/employer representation. Employees should be able to participate in health and safety matters without fear of subsequent retaliation. Whilst the law does not provide general protection for whistleblowing employees, dismissal for involvement in health and safety matters is deemed to be unfair (S100 Employment Rights Act 1996).

Back injuries are a particular source of concern for the nurse. Handling heavy patients leads to the risk of back strain. Guidance is given in the *Manual Handling Regulations* (1992) (SI 1992 No. 2793) as to measures which should be taken to safeguard the position of the nurse. Guidance has also been issued on this matter by the Health and Safety Executive. The regulations require that, wherever possible, hazardous manual handling by employees should be avoided (reg. 4(1)(a)). Where it cannot be avoided the risks of manual handling should be the subject of assessment (reg. 4(1)(b)). Appropriate measures should be taken to reduce the risk of injury (reg. 4(1)(b)(ii)). Information should be given as to the risk of each load. This assessment should be reviewed if there is reason to believe that it is outdated (reg. 4(2)). Nurses should be given training as to dealing with loads.

The area of health and safety raises a multitude of other issues. These are the subject of a book in themselves and the nurse wishing to gain a more specialist knowledge is referred to other texts on the subject (Smith and Thomas, 1996iii; Morris and Archer, 1993). Particular issues in relation to employer's liability in common law and for breach of statutory duty to the injured nurse or patient are explored below.

Suitability to be a nurse

Many employers undertake screening programmes before they employ new staff. It is important that an employee possesses the necessary qualities for a particular job. Suitability for employment is, of course, of paramount importance in the context of health care provision. It is important to ensure that prospective nurses are suited to the work and that they themselves will not present any risk of harm to the patient.

A graphic illustration of the importance of monitoring those who care for patients was provided by the Beverley Allitt case (DOH, 1991). A number of children died at Grantham General Hospital and others were harmed. The incidents were traced back to a nurse, Beverley Allitt, who had been employed at the hospital. She was eventually tried and convicted of murder, attempted murder and causing grievous bodily harm. During the trial, evidence was given to the effect that she had developed the condition Munchausen's syndrome by proxy.

Following the incident, an enquiry was established under Sir Cecil Clothier (News, 1994). The Clothier report recommended that a person with evidence of a major personality disorder should not be employed as a nurse. It was suggested that after qualifying and obtaining their first post, nurses should undergo formal health screening. In addition, procedures for management referrals to occupational health should make clear the criteria which will trigger such referrals. The Clothier report also recommended that consideration should be given as to how general practitioners might, with a job applicant's consent, be asked to certify that there is nothing in his or her medical history which would make the person unsuitable for employment in the NHS.

The National Health and Safety Executive issued a circular giving guidance as to procedures which should be undertaken to check possible criminal backgrounds of persons who apply for posts giving substantial access to children (HSG(94)43). Such checks are particularly appropriate for posts in which there is unsupervised access to children requiring lengthy in-patient care. The circular suggests that the checks should include both national and local police records.

There has been some concern expressed regarding these guidelines and subsequent guidelines issued by the RCN (RCN, 1995) and as to vetting generally as it may amount to a 'witch hunt'. Nursing employers have to tread a difficult path when safeguarding the interests of patients and other staff, while at the same time not hounding employees and totally limiting the employment prospects of persons who may have suffered temporary difficulties (Naish, 1995).

Screening and testing for HIV and Hepatitis B

Particular controversy surrounds the management of health care professionals who test HIV positive. The UKCC (1993a) recommends that if nurses believe that they are infected with HIV they should obtain specialist medical advice as to what are acceptable areas of practice and that failure to do so would be to contravene the Code of Conduct. It advises that a nurse who is HIV positive should not continue to practice in a post involving 'contact with sharp instruments, sharp splinters or edges of bone, particularly where the hands are not completely visible'. In addition, a nurse who believes that another nurse is HIV positive and is potentially placing patients at risk, needs to consider very carefully her or his obligations under the professional code (see Appendix 1). The fact that a nurse is confirmed as HIV positive is not by itself grounds for automatic dismissal from her or his post; rather, it should lead to a reconsideration of the nurse's role.

What if an NHS Trust tells a nurse that s/he should be tested to determine HIV status? Pre-employment testing has been upheld as lawful (*X* v. *Commission of the European Communities* [1995] IRLR 320). As far as employees in post are concerned, the Court of Appeal has stated that employees shall not be required to submit to a medical examination unless there is a reasonable basis for the belief that they are suffering from a physical or mental disability which would cause harm to patients or that it would harm the quality of treatment provided (*Bliss* v. *SE Thames RHA* [1985] 1 RPC 308). It should be noted that the *Midwives Rules* (UKCC, 1993b) state that a practising midwife should allow herself to undergo a medical examination if this is necessary and it has been requested by the local supervising authority.

The risk of transmission of HIV by nurses to patients is very low and there are no instances of this having occurred in England and Wales. There is a greater risk of transmission of other infectious diseases such as hepatitis B. Nurses who know/suspect that they are, for example, a carrier of such a condition should be aware of the legal implications should they continue to practice in situations in which they may place patients at risk of harm. In 1995 a surgeon, Dr Gaud, was prosecuted for the common law offence of public nuisance because he performed or assisted in the performance of surgery when knowing that he was a carrier of hepatitis B (Mulholland, 1995). Dr Gaud knew that he was carrying a highly infectious strain of the virus but still went ahead and operated. The nurse should be aware of guidance issued on this subject by the Department of Health (DOH, 1993). Failure to follow such guidance may also result in civil liability and in the nurse being sued by a patient who contracts the illness from the nurse. For a nurse to proceed knowing that she was infected and not to inform the patient of that fact would amount to vitiation of any consent to the treatment procedure which the patient had given (Wright, 1997).

The Department of Health has issued guidance to the effect that health care workers who are at risk of contracting hepatitis B should be offered vaccination (Kloss, 1995; DOH, 1993). Employers should monitor responses to the vaccine. If health care professionals who are working in 'exposure prone' procedures have what is an abnormal response to the vaccine, then they should be removed from that work. Also carriers of hepatitis B who are e-antigen positive should desist in carrying out procedures where there is a risk that if they e.g. suffer a needlstick injury they may contaminate a patient. Vaccination and follow-up tests are voluntary (DOH, 1993i). It should be noted that the guidance states that if health professionals are aware that other health professionals are not complying with the guidance then they should inform the appropriate authorities (DOH, 1993ii). If a Trust, for example, does not follow this guidance and a patient is infected by hepatitis B from a health care worker, then this may lead to legal proceedings being brought by the infected patient against the trust.

A nurse, as a patient, is entitled to respect for the confidentiality of her health information. However, there may be instances in which a trust decides to go public regarding the health of a nurse. This may arise in a situation in which it was believed that patients may have been at risk of infection from the nurse. While public disclosure of the medical history of individual health professionals diagnosed as being HIV positive or having developed AIDS has taken place in the context of surgeons and obstetricians, it is questionable whether it would generally be justifiable to reveal publicly such information in the case of a nurse. This is because, in all but the most exceptional situations, nurses are unlikely to be in a position in which blood/bodily fluids are passed to a patient.

If a nurse falls ill, this may ultimately constitute a basis for dismissal by the nurse's employer. Whether dismissal on the basis of ill health is justifiable relates to the individual circumstances of the particular case (*East Lindsay DC* v. *Daubney* [1977] ICR 566). Relevant factors would include the circumstances of the nurse in question, the length of time s/he has been and is likely to be absent from work and the urgency with which a replacement is required.

Liability for unsafe conditions at work

Occupier's liability

A nurse falls on uneven flooring in the hospital and injures her back. Workmen are in the process of repairing part of the floor where the flooring had become cracked but overnight left a section of the floor uncovered and unmarked and the nurse stumbled on it. She suffers bruising and a cracked elbow. In such a situation an action may be brought against the hospital under the Occupier's Liability Act 1957. This Act imposes obligations upon 'occupiers' - persons with some degree of control associated with/arising from their activities on the premises. The Act covers structural defects and other hazards which have arisen due to the state of the premises. The duty imposed is:

> 'a duty to take such care as in all the circumstances of the case is reasonable to see that the visitor will be reasonably safe in using the premises for the purpose for which he is invited or permitted by the occupier to be there.(s2(2))'

This duty would fall on the Trust. Occupiers need to take care to avoid harm and make persons aware of the risk, particularly in the case of children. (The 1957 Act requires that occupiers must take into account the fact that children are less careful than adults (s2(3) Occupier Liability Act 1957).) The obligation under the statute may be discharged if a warning notice has been put up stating, 'Warning - floor is being repaired - proceed with care' (s2(4)(a) Occupier's Liability Act 1957). However, simply putting up a notice does not provide automatic protection for an occupier. The warning must be such as to allow the person to be reasonably safe. A notice may not provide sufficient warning if it is too small or if it is not immediately obvious or if those using the area are unable to read it or heed it.

Duty to ensure a safe system of work

If the nurse is injured in the workplace then s/he may bring a claim for compensation for harm suffered against her employer. A nurse may bring a claim in negligence. For an action in negligence to be brought it must be shown that there was a breach of the duty owed to the employee and that damage flowed from this breach of duty. If there has been a breach of a duty owed to an employee under statute then it is sufficient show that the breach of statutory duty was a material cause of the injury suffered.

Breaches of the Health and Safety at Work Act 1974 do not entitle a person to bring damages in a civil court (s47, 1974 Act), but breaches of health and safety regulations may lead to a cause of action. At common law, employers are under a duty to take reasonable care to ensure their employees' safety. There is a duty to ensure that the premises themselves are safe and that there is a safe means of access (*Latimer* v. *AEC Ltd* [1953] AC 643). There is an obligation to establish a safe system of work and to ensure that it is correctly operated (*McDermid* v. *Nash Dredging* [1987] 2 All ER 878 HL).

A nurse is severely injured when a hoist breaks and a patient falls on to her. In addition to an action on the basis that the trust owes her a duty to provide a safe system of work, which also includes an obligation to provide employees with proper plant and equipment, there is also an obligation under statute. The Employer's Liability (Defective Equipment) Act 1969 states that an employer is liable to an employee who suffers personal injury during the course of employment as a result of a defect in the equipment provided by his employer. The Trust is liable even if the defect is wholly or partly attributable to the fault of a third party. A Trust would not, however, be liable if the nurse was not making proper use of the equipment provided, for example if she had not been operating the hoist properly (*Parkinson* v. *Lyle Shipping Co.* [1964] 2 *Lloyds Reports* 79). If the nurse has contributed through her own conduct to harm suffered this may lead to a reduction in damages (S1(1) Law Reform Contributory Negligence Act 1945).

Poor working conditions and harm to health - stress at work

The obligation of an employer to provide a safe system of work applies not only to the employees' physical health but also to their mental health. Nursing is a demanding profession and certain aspects of health care are particularly stressful. A nurse who falls ill and claims that this was caused by unduly high stress levels in the workplace may bring legal proceedings claiming compensation for the harm suffered.

The fact that a contract of employment may stipulate stressful working conditions does not by itself mean that a nurse who suffers physical or psychological harm consequent upon that stress cannot bring a claim for damages. This was made clear by the case of *Johnston* v. *Bloomsbury*

AHA ([1991] 2 All ER 293). Here, a junior hospital doctor brought an action claiming that his employer had broken an implied duty to take reasonable care for his safety and had broken his contract of employment. He was required by his contract to work a basic week of 40 hours and to be available for up to 48 hours per week overtime. In the Court of Appeal a majority of the judges held that he had an arguable case. Stuart Smith L.J. held that the health authority was under a duty to provide a safe system of work. While the obligation to work up to 88 hours per week was contained in a junior doctor's contract, this had to be set against an employer's duty to take reasonable care for the employee's safety.

One difficulty in bringing such actions is that of showing that stress-induced psychiatric injury is foreseeable. Much depends on the circumstances of the individual case. In some instances employers can justifiably argue that they were not aware that their employee had been subject to what were excessive stress levels. Where an employer is, however, put on notice that an employee is susceptible to such a breakdown and then that employee returns to work and suffers a second nervous breakdown due to stressful working conditions, then an action consequent upon the second breakdown may meet with more success (*Walker* v. *Northumbria County Council* [1995] 1 All ER 737). A nurse would also have to establish that it was the stressful working conditions themselves which amounted to a material cause of her or his breakdown. This may itself be problematic; in many situations stress levels are influenced by factors external to the employment relationship itself, such as home and family life. It is also the case that the assessment of stress levels is a matter which would fall under the employee obligations under the Health and Safety at Work Act 1974 and the Management of Health and Safety at Work Regulations 1992.

Product liability

If a nurse is injured when a piece of equipment she is using fractures, s/he may bring an action claiming damages for the harm suffered under the Consumer Protection Act 1987. This statute allows an action to be brought against producers and suppliers of defective products where the defect in the product led to damage. The legislation introduced following a European Convention on Products liability can potentially be also used by patients e.g. if harmed by defective drugs. Guidance issued within the NHS as to the operation of the legislation states that a health authority may be liable under the 1987 Act in a number of situations (HN(88)3, HN(FP)(88)5). First, they may be liable as a producer of medicines, appliances or pharmaceutical products. Second, they may be liable unless the producer or supplier can be identified. Finally, they may be liable as a 'keeper' if the supplier or producer shows that the product has not been used according to instructions or not sufficiently maintained.

The important difference between the 1987 Act and a negligence action at common law, as outlined in Chapter 2, is that fault does not have to be shown. It is sufficient to establish that the defect *caused* the damage. In considering what amounts to a defect, section 3(2) outlines a number of factors to be taken into account:

> 'the manner in which, and the purposes for which, the product has been marketed, its get-up, the use of any mark in relation to the product and any instructions for, or warnings with respect to, doing or refraining from doing anything with or in relation to the product.'

If the injured nurse had, for example, not followed the instructions then she could not bring an action under the statute.

An action may only be brought against a producer of the product within 10 years of the product having been supplied. There is a defence to actions under the legislation if, at the time the product was produced, scientific and technical knowledge was not such that:

> 'a producer of products of the same description as the product in question might have been expected to have discovered the defect. (s4(1))'

While use of this statute remains theoretically possible, establishing liability may be difficult practically. The fact that the product is defective needs to be shown, which can be as difficult as establishing negligence in a standard common law claim (see Jones, 1996).

Criminal injuries compensation

A nurse on duty in accident and emergency is injured when a patient turns violent and assaults both patients and staff. This may result in the patient being prosecuted in criminal law for the injury given to the nurse. In addition, the nurse may bring a claim for compensation for her or his injuries under the Criminal Injuries Compensation Scheme (Criminal Injuries Compensation Act 1995). Claims can be made under this scheme where injury has been caused by a crime of violence, when apprehending an offender or suspected offender, or stopping a criminal offence. Claims are made to the Criminal Injuries Compensation Authority.

In order to succeed in the claim the nurse must show that s/he suffered disease, or harm to her physical or mental condition, or, if pregnant, to the pregnancy. The person bringing a claim under the scheme does not have to show that the person who inflicted the injury has been convicted in a criminal court but s/he must show that s/he has taken reasonable steps within a reasonable time to inform the police or the appropriate authorities.

Awards made under the scheme are usually in the form of a lump sum along the lines of the awards of damages made in tort cases. However, a person who has been injured may submit a further claim if, since the previous award was made, the injury has deteriorated and it would be unjust not to award a further sum. If a civil court has already awarded damages against the person who has attacked the nurse then this sum is deducted from any award which s/he may receive from the Criminal Injuries Compensation Scheme. If s/he decides to bring a civil action for damages against the attacker after an award has been made under the Compensation Scheme and is successful, s/he must repay the Authority from the damages awarded. This is to ensure that s/he is not doubly compensated. Sums are paid in accordance with a tariff of standard sums with regard to various types of injury. There is provision for some adjustment to the injury to take account of its severity.

References

Criminal Injuries Compensation Authority (1996) *Guide to the Criminal Injuries Compensation Scheme*.

Deakin, S. and Morris, G. (1995) *Labour Law*, Butterworths, London.

Department of Health (1994) 'Disclosure to NHS employers of criminal background of those with access to children.' *Health Service Guidelines*, **43**(94), September. HMSO, London.

Department of Health (1993) Protecting health care workers and patients from hepatitis B. *Health Service Guidelines*, **40** (93). HMSO, London, (i) para 5.5; (ii) para 5.6.

Department of Health (1991) *Report of the independent inquiry relating to the deaths and injuries on the childrens ward at Grantham and Kestevin General Hospital during the period February to April 1991.* HMSO, London.

Du-Fen, V. and Warnock, O. (1995) *Employment Law in the NHS*. Cavendish Publishers, London.

Health and Safety Executive (1989) Health and Safety Information for Employees Regulations. HSE.

Jones, M. (1996) *Textbook on Torts*. Blackstones, London, para 10.2.

Kloss, D. (1995) *Occupational Health Law* (2nd edn), Blackwells Scientific, Oxford.

Morris and Archer (1993) *Trade Unions, Employers and the Law*, 2nd edn.

Mulholland, M. (1995) 'Public nuisance: a new use for an old tool.' *Professional Negligence*, **11**, 700.

Naish, J. (1995) 'Can another Beverley Allit be stopped from preying on patients.' *Health Care Risk Report,* **12**.

News (1994) 'News; Clothier inquiry criticises OH.' *Occupational Health*, **74**, (March).

RCN (1995) *Health Assessment: advice to managers*. RCN, London.

Smith, I. and Thomas, G. (1996) *Smith and Woods Industrial Law*. Butterworths, London, (i) pp. 231-260; (ii) Chapter 10; (iii) Chapter 13.

UKCC (1993a) Registrar's letter. Annexe 1, para 17, 6 April. United Kingdom Central Council for Nursing, Midwifery and Health Visiting, London.

UKCC (1993b) Midwives Rules. United Kingdom Central Council for Nursing, Midwifery and Health Visiting, London, No. 39.

Wright, M. (1997) 'Health-care workers and HIV screening: pragmatism or public interest?' *Journal of Social Welfare and Family Law*, 17.

Chapter 10

Litigation

John Peysner

Introduction

It is currently fashionable to say that civil litigation is 'out of control', with costs and damages increasing unreasonably. Litigation has grown for a number of reasons. Since the late 1960s governments have placed emphasis on rights and responsibilities being expressed in an individual rather than a collective form. Legislation introduced includes anti-discrimination laws in the fields of racial and sexual discrimination, protection against unfair dismissal or redundancy and a range of measures to protect health and safety at work. It seems likely that the expanded role of the European Union in our law will continue this trend. Enforcement of these rights is largely through tribunals or, in the field of accidents at work, the civil courts (see Chapter 1). The emphasis on 'individualism' has also created an environment where consumers of goods or services are less reticent than formerly in demanding compensation and individuals, injured as they go about their daily life, more prepared to bring a claim.

As explained in Chapters 2 and 3, there has been an increase in negligence litigation and in complaints. In 1947, as the NHS began, it faced only 49 clinical negligence claims and by 1957 it was still only 92 (*Nursing Times*, 1994). From the 1980s the number of clinical negligence cases and their associated costs grew rapidly. Within the area of clinical negligence, the Medical Defence Union in 1994 reported a 15% annual increase in malpractice claims (*The Guardian*, 31 May 1994). The Legal Aid Board reported that 11,667 legal aid certificates were granted in 1992–93 to pursue 'clinical negligence' compared with 18,658 in 1991–92 and 8870 in 1990–91. The Department of Health estimated the annual cost to health authorities of meeting negligence claims was £53 million (1990–91), £80 million (1991–92),and £125 million (1993–94) (*Health Service Journal*, 1994). This compares with an estimate of £9.3 million as compensation for losses to health authorities in 1986–87 (Bowles and Jones, 1990). Latest estimates suggest that the total cost of NHS clinical negligence is around

£200 million and is likely to grow at around 25% over the 5-year period from 1996, of which the share borne by trusts will rise from about 10% to 75%.

It is clear that payment of damages of this order, together with the legal, managerial and staff time involved in dealing with this volume of litigation, is having an increasing impact on the resources available for health care. What are the causes of this rise in clinical accident litigation? It seems inherently unlikely that health professionals became less skilful during the period. One influential factor is the growth of consumerism in the UK, with an increasingly questioning attitude to authority and organisations. A key development was the emergence of the patient's consumer group Action for the Victims of Medical Accidents (AVMA) in 1982. Patients are less prepared to accept health workers' views without questioning them and many feel that someone must be to blame for an unsatisfactory outcome.

As the demand for compensation has multiplied, the number of lawyers skilled in this type of work has also increased. The individual citizen also has greater awareness of his or her rights and is more willing to enforce these rights through the courts, bringing local and central government and other organisations (including the NHS) to account for failure to provide proper services or for making ill-judged decisions in fields as diverse as environmental protection, education and benefits. It is not surprising that individual nurses, in particular those employed by the NHS with its vast, complex organisation, will become involved in many aspects of litigation.

This chapter considers the litigation process from a practical perspective. It considers the involvement of nurses in cases, in tribunals and courts in relation to their professional activity. Chapter 1 considered the essential difference between a criminal and civil case but, as mentioned above, nurses should be reassured that involvement by them in criminal litigation arising out of their work is, in practice, extremely rare. Within the scope of this chapter it is not possible to discuss the practical impact on a nurse of the many and varied ways in which s/he could be involved in the litigation process (see Chapter 1). A number of general issues are explored through case studies at the end of the chapter. The first case study deals with an allegation of clinical negligence by a nurse. The second case study deals with a civil claim brought by a nurse arising out of an accident. There follows a short discussion about some criminal issues. By nurses understanding the process of litigation, by seeking prompt and efficient advice, and by acting appropriately to manage risk, they can effectively protect themselves against the threat of litigation.

Litigation process - the involvement of the nurse

In outline, the litigation system that faces the nurse can be broken down as follows:

Bringing a case in court

If a nurse is injured at work, perhaps in a moving and handling accident, then the nurse would bring a claim - would *sue* - as a *plaintiff* and the trust, or other employer, would be the *defendant.*

Facing a case in court

If a nurse were alleged to have damaged a patient by a clinical error then, in theory, the patient would be the *plaintiff* and the nurse the *defendant.* In fact, as explained in Chapter 2, because of the operation of vicarious liability it would be very unusual for a nurse to be a party to litigation in such circumstances. An action would usually be brought against the nurse's employer.

Bringing a case before an industrial tribunal

If a nurse claims to have been racially discriminated against, or unfairly dismissed, then the nurse is the *applicant* in the case - the *application*, and the employer is the *respondent.*

Being brought before a professional body

A nurse may be called to account by the professional body which controls the nurse's right to work; for example the United Kingdom Central Council for Nursing, Midwifery and Health Visiting (UKCC). This could involve the nurse being a *respondent* to an application to remove her from the register.

Being a witness

A nurse may not be involved as a party to litigation but may be a witness called to give evidence on behalf of a party (normally, assisting the nurse's employer).

A nurse may be involved with more than one of these areas at once:

Example 1

A nurse suffers a serious radiation injury when using defective equipment supplied to a trust by a manufacturer. The nurse may sue the trust for failing to provide a safe system of work and the manufacturer for producing a defective product. The nurse may be a witness for the Health and Safety Executive in a prosecution brought against both the trust and the manufacturer.

Example 2

A practice nurse receives a telephone call from a private nursing home which wishes to employ one of the practice's patients as a care assistant, subject to a satisfactory clinical reference. Contrary to the rules of the practice, the nurse gives details of the patient's clinical history over the phone. Unfortunately, the nurse picks up the wrong card and gives the history of an entirely different patient who happens to be HIV positive. The nursing home withdraws the job offer. The nurse may face an action for breach of confidence, or defamation from the patient and may end up being dismissed from the practice's employment (see Chapter 9). Whilst the dismissal could be challenged in an industrial tribunal, the nurse might face the possibility of disciplinary proceedings by the UKCC for breaching patient confidentiality.

Burden and standard of proof

To establish a legal claim the burden of proof must be satisfied, as explained in Chapter 2. In a civil case the *burden* lies on the person bringing the claim. In Example 1 above the nurse must prove negligence by the trust. The *standard of proof* in such a case is on the balance of probabilities, i.e. the nurse must show that it is *more likely than not* that the trust was negligent. In a clinical negligence case the patient must show that the trust was negligent in the health care provided, on a balance of probabilities. In contrast, other types of cases have different burdens and standards. For example, to prove a criminal case the prosecuting authorities must establish the defendant's guilt 'beyond reasonable doubt', which is a much higher standard; in deciding if a nurse should be sacked for misconduct a trust disciplinary board may only act on reasonable suspicion, which is a much lower standard.

How your legal duty to take care may involve you in litigation - will you be sued?

A National Health Service patient whether of a trust, GP fund holder, health authority or non-fundholding GP does not contract personally with the health provider. Instead, the provider and staff offer a service on a statutory basis. In the private sector, patients (or their families) make a contract with the hospital and if this is broken, e.g. by a failure to take reasonable care, then they may be able to sue for damages for breach of contract. It is also unlikely for an individual nurse in the NHS to have a contractual relationship with an individual patient. Instead, a contract is usually made with the health provider, not an individual member of staff.

Even though there is no contract, a nurse may be at risk of an action in negligence. Generally, the patient has a choice: to sue the nurse and/or the employer. This is because the employer, whether in the private or public sector, is normally responsible for the negligent actions of the nurse. As explained in Chapter 2, vicarious liability is present in every case except where the nurse has acted so far beyond contract as to be acting 'on a frolic of his or her own'. However, it is possible. In Example 2 above, if the practice nurse has been properly trained and the surgery's rules on confidentiality are clear, then it could be said that any liability rests only on the nurse and not the practice. Patients will, usually, be content not to sue a nurse as well as an employer. Damages can only be recovered once and if the claim succeeds against the employer, who has the deepest pocket, then there is little point in increasing the costs and complexity of the proceedings by adding the nurse as a party. (Naturally, the employer would require the nurse to cooperate in the defence of the claim.)

On the rare occasion when the employer disclaims vicarious responsibility, a nurse carrying out private practice work may be sued personally. In these situations the nurse is not acting on behalf of another; no vicarious liability applies. To ensure that nurses are protected, they must obtain adequate insurance cover and access to legal advice.

Damages in clinical negligence cases

One area of concern in clinical negligence cases is the perception that the amount - the quantum - of damages awarded in such cases is escalating out of control. For reasons explained below, this impression is not correct; but in order to appreciate this, it is important to understand the basis on which a plaintiff's damages are assessed. It is not possible in the limited space of this chapter to give a complete description of every aspect that goes to make up a financial claim for personal injury. (The same rules apply whether the claim is for an injury to a patient caused by clinical negligence - a medical accident - or an ordinary accident at work to a nurse.) The basic rule is that the victim should be put back in the same position as s/he was before the accident happened.

General damages

If a patient is a victim of a negligent medical accident, then as well as compensation for any immediate pain and suffering, a claim may be brought for 'general damages'. These represent the difference between the patient's *expected* outcome following treatment and his or her *actual* outcome. This difference - called loss of amenity - is based on expert evidence presented to the court. For example, a young woman is admitted to hospital with a fractured right leg. The casualty officer sets it badly. The patient might have expected to resume normal life on recovery with a full range of activity, including sporting and leisure pursuits; in fact , she has a permanent limp. General damages represent a money figure to compensate for this loss. If the same bad setting happened to an ill geriatric patient, then damages would be assessed on the more limited outcome expected from an old, ill patient.

How are these different factors calculated? The baseline is a set of generally recognised conventional figures for specific types of injury. The judge then takes into account individual factors of pain and suffering and loss of amenity, relying on published reports of similar cases. This process is more art than science, but in general results in awards that are relatively low. For example, a fracture in an older patient might be valued at less than £6000. Currently the highest award of general damages recommended by the Judicial Studies Board for an injury of maximum severity, e.g. tetraplegia with pain and the awareness of pain is £125,000 (Judicial Studies Board, 1996). This book is available to every judge deciding a case and gives helpful but not binding guidelines. In view of this, why is there a perception that clinical negligence damages are very high and increasing out of control? The answer lies in the additional factors making up the overall award which are detailed below.

Loss of earnings, earning power and congenial employment

Before her accident the young woman in our example was employed as a hairdresser. She was highly talented and relatively well paid. She is now unable to stand all day and works in a supermarket as a checkout operator at a lower wage. How is she compensated? Her loss of wages is calculated by taking her annual loss (the difference between her net wages as a shop assistant and a hairdresser) and multiplying it by a figure - the *multiplier* - which represents the years left before she would have retired from hairdressing. Calculating the multiplier is not an exact science; the judge would decide having heard argument from both sides. If she would normally have worked until 60 years of age and the accident happened at 20, then her income may be restricted for 40 years. However, the calculation must take into account the possibility that her career might have been shortened anyway; by child care, or occupational problems such as varicose veins. Furthermore, by getting her loss of earnings in a lump sum at 20 years of age rather than having to earn it over a long period, she can invest it and earn interest. These factors reduce the multiplier, in this case to perhaps 18 years. The court then takes into account her loss of earning power, that is, her future job security. Let us imagine that her injuries were not so serious as to cause her to give up hairdressing but, in the future, she might have difficulties in changing her job, because of her disability. She would be entitled to an extra sum of money for this disadvantage in the labour market. She may also be entitled to an extra sum for ' loss of enjoyment of employment', a special award available to policemen, firemen, nurses, etc., reflecting the total commitment and camaraderie of their jobs.

Future expenses and interest

Our patient may also have additional expenses, such as physiotherapy, which must be taken into account. Any expenses actually incurred before a settlement or trial, e.g. taxi fares to hospital, damaged clothing, etc. (called special damage) would also be paid. The whole amount of general damages, special damages and expenses would have added to it interest from the date of the medical accident to the date the damages are paid.

Mitigating loss

After a disabling accident the patient cannot simply rely on the defendant to support her. In our example if the patient refused to take alternative employment, perhaps because it was not paid enough, then she could be held to have not mitigated her loss. She would be unable to recover all her loss of earnings, but only the difference between her loss as a hairdresser and an amount representing a job she could do, for example, shop work.

Benefits

Following the accident a patient would normally receive state benefits. These would be taken into account and reduce the damages. The defendant would hold back an amount equal to the benefits paid and pay this to the state.

Catastrophic injuries and structured settlements

The example outlined above would attract quite modest damages. However, in some cases the damages are much higher and it is these relatively rare cases which hit the headlines. Take a brain-damaged baby. While such an infant may have a relatively normal expectation of life, s/he would require constant nursery care and the provision of expensive specialist equipment for movement, communication and entertainment, all of which would need regular replacement. These elements of loss, taken over such a long period, despite a discount for early payment, can produce huge awards - £1 million and more. In the case of a tetraplegic adult again, medical science has advanced the average life expectancy of such patients, who need constant care and cannot earn their living. If a patient was a successful business person or highly paid employee then loss of earnings, together with the cost of buying or adopting a suitable home and staffing it, can add up to a huge award.

The system of paying such awards of damages in a lump sum is increasingly seen to be unsatisfactory. It has major cash flow implications for a trust and may leave a patient vulnerable if inflation rises faster than expected or the patient lives longer than expected. One method of resolving this problem is to create what is known as a 'structured settlement'. Having calculated the total damages part, it is then paid over to meet the patient's immediate needs, and the balance is normally invested in a tax efficient annuity which produces a stream of income during the whole of the patient's life, index linked to inflation. The NHS is increasingly encouraging the use of structured settlements which are funded by the Department of Health and Treasury rather than through an annuity.

Who pays for clinical negligence?

Prior to 1991 doctors (and dentists) in the hospital service were *separately* responsible for their own actions, though their own clinical defence organisations, in return for subscriptions paid by the doctors, organised legal defence and paid the damages and legal costs of members involved in clinical negligence actions. The liability of nurses rested directly with the health authorities, who were at that time providing hospital services. Where clinical accidents arise from errors or omissions in the operating theatre, the failure to diagnose, or the iatrogenic effect of drugs, the source of liability or information has historically rested within the clinical rather than the nursing staff. There has always been the exception of midwives who, as a consequence of their role, were at risk of litigation.

Since 1991, the introduction of Crown indemnity (now trust indemnity) has assimilated the position of clinical and nursing staff; both can normally rely on the trust, or the remaining clinical health authorities, to provide 'cover' through the mechanism of vicarious liability and solicitors acting for the trust would expect cooperation from and would extend support to all staff, whether clinical or nursing, involved in a clinical negligence case. The mechanics of such claims are explored further in Chapter 2.

Indemnity and insurance

As explained in Chapter 2, the health provider would, normally, be vicariously responsible for the alleged negligence of a nurse. This doctrine ensures that the negligently injured victim does not have to worry about showing whether the nurse alone or, perhaps, the trust managers were at fault; recovery against either would be paid by the trust. However, in the law of negligence there is a right of indemnity for the employer; damages paid out to a patient can potentially be recovered from the individual health worker. There is no legal bar to an attempted recovery by way of indemnity from a nurse, but there are profound practical difficulties. Firstly, it would curtail the policy objective of increasing the competencies and role of nurses. Secondly, it would force nurses to increase their insurance cover, creating a fresh funding crisis. For this reason, the Department of Health has discouraged moves to enforce indemnities.

Nurses who are employed by GP practices or private hospitals will not necessarily benefit from this approach. In principle, they could be involved in litigation as defendants, although most plaintiffs would prefer to bring an action against the GP or the hospital. The attitude of the GP or hospital to seeking an indemnity will vary, and thus nurses should ensure that they are adequately insured.

Importance of records

A health provider may have a perfectly viable defence to an allegation of clinical negligence, but without adequate records it would be virtually impossible to defend the case. In clinical work, it is almost inevitable that staff will forget the details of individual patients. The nurse who counts the swabs makes a note as the count proceeds, otherwise as time passes s/he will have no recollection of the number retained and whether it is time to start fishing around in the abdomen to find the missing one. The doctor who takes a consent from a patient for a dilation and curettage gets the patient to sign a consent form otherwise, in the course of a busy day, there is a risk that the doctor would forget what conversation s/he had with the patient and whether proper consent was obtained.

One difficulty is that most medico-legal litigation relates to clinical accidents which, in themselves, are neither dramatic nor particularly memorable. If a surgeon carries out an amputation on the wrong limb and this is discovered immediately after the operation, then the events would be permanently imprinted in the minds of the whole surgical team and, no doubt, the health provider's staff and lawyers would immediately take statements from all involved. However, allegations of clinical negligence often relate to a series of interlocking decisions by a number of health professionals over a period of days; each decision may have seemed innocuous, only the overall picture may reveal an impression of poor clinical care. In such circumstances it is inevitable that potential witnesses, often including the patient, would have no useful memory of the events. This illustrates the importance of accurate records.

However, in practice, it appears that records are often inaccurate. An Audit Commission report based on examining records in some 40 hospitals identified that 30% of doctors' notes (history sheets) were not legible, accurate, timely and comprehensive; 20% of prescription sheets were illegible; 40% of hand-written discharge medication sheets were illegible and 90% of discharge summaries contained no reference to any information given to the patient or relatives (Audit Commission, 1995a). Inaccurate records can cause great difficulties. Whilst there is some reason to think that nurse records are better kept than clinical records (particularly those of junior clinical staff), there is no room for complacency in this area.

Judges are unlikely to be critical of records which make a fair attempt to record matters of clinical importance and which omit matters which 'at the time' were of less relevance. The patient's advisors can then see, from the start, if proper care has been taken, rather than having to wait until the attending doctor's statement is made available in the course of the litigation process. The UKCC (1993) states that the record:

'14.1 ...is directed primarily to serving the interests and care of the patient or client to whom the record relates and enabling the provision of care, the prevention of disease and the promotion of care, the prevention of disease and the promotion of health and

14.2 will demonstrate the chronology of events and all significant consultations, assessments, observations, decisions, interventions and outcomes.'

They go on to note that, in addition to the primary purpose of serving the interests of the patient, a record may have legal implications. They state that the records should provide:

'22.1 a comprehensive picture of care delivered, associated outcomes and other relevant information;
22.1 pertinent information about the condition of the patient or client at any given time and the measures taken to respond to identified need;
22.3 evidence that the practitioner's common law duty of care has been understood and honoured; and
22.4 a record of the arrangements made for the continuity of a patient's care on discharge from hospital.'

Obtaining records for litigation

General issues relating to confidentiality and confidentiality of records are dealt with in Chapter 7. The present section deals with access to health records in the context of civil litigation. The Access to Health Records Act 1990 gives patients rights of access to health records compiled after November 1991. (A patient is also entitled to any computerised health records created after November 1987 by virtue of the Data Protection Act 1984.) Both Acts contain similar provisions which limit access in specific circumstances, e.g. where the information contained in the records is likely to cause serious harm to the patient. This could cover a situation where doctors have not given the patient a frank diagnosis of a possibly terminal condition, for fear that the patient will 'give up the struggle'. In practice, limitations on disclosure under the Act are normally restricted to psychiatric records.

Pre-proceedings discovery

If the patient seeks records prior to 1991, or believes that the records offered are incomplete, then court action may be taken to obtain full records. Normally, a party to a court case is only entitled to see the relevant documents held by his or her opponent after proceedings have started: this legal process is called *discovery*. However, in clinical negligence cases plaintiffs can apply for copies of records held by a trust which they wish to use in a forthcoming case. Some documents are unobtainable, they are covered by what is called 'legal professional privilege' because they relate to communications between lawyer and client or were created because of a possible claim. Virtually all records specific to a patient, including clinical findings, the results of tests and records of any consent given would have to be produced - their dominant purpose was not for the investigation and defence of a legal claim. But what about less obviously clinical material? What if a patient's case is the subject of a confidential Department of Health enquiry (such as a perinatal death enquiry)? It depends on the 'dominant purpose' for holding the enquiry: to establish the truth or as a preliminary step to seeking legal advice. The decision would depend upon the facts of a particular case and, on occasion, public policy considerations.

Role of expert opinion

Some clinical negligence cases are tried on the facts alone; for example, it is agreed by all parties that before procedure A the nurse should carry out test B. The nurse claims to have done so but there is no record and the patient denies that the test was carried out. Many cases involve a dispute as to the correct approach, with experts arguing as to the appropriateness of the practice. As explained in Chapter 2, to win such a case the plaintiff would normally have to show that the actions of the nurse were not in accord with a responsible body of professional nursing opinion and for this she would need expert clinical opinion. Increasingly, this will be informed by relevant protocols and guidelines (see Chapter 4).

EXAMPLE: A further role of expert opinion is in relation to *causation*. As explained in Chapter 2, to succeed in an action for negligence the plaintiff must not only establish negligence, but that the negligence has caused the damage complained of. This is often a very difficult task and as stated in Chapter 2, many claims fall; whilst negligence is established, causation is in dispute.

A patient has a routine scan for breast cancer. The technician misses a tumour and the patient dies. An expert in scanning techniques considering the case for the health provider establishes that an operator error has occurred and that this was negligent. However, this would not be the end of the story. The case notes would also be passed to a surgeon specialising in the care and treatment of patients with breast cancer. That second surgeon may establish that at the time of the scan the deceased was suffering from an aggressive, metastasising tumour, which even if detected would not have been operable: the error has not led to any damage; the course of the patient's disease was inevitable.

In establishing negligence there must be a statement of the relevant body or bodies of clinical knowledge, both in terms of the literature and of actual clinical practice. Experts called in clinical negligence cases tend to be leaders in their field, impartially available to plaintiffs and defendants alike and currently in practice or recently retired. An expert should report only in areas where s/he has genuine expertise. For example, a GP could be an expert witness on GP practice; to call a GP to give evidence on nursing practice would be inappropriate. Equally, a general nurse should judge another general nurse, not a nurse practitioner expert.

Risk management environment and the defence of clinical negligence claims

The discussion above concerning clinical negligence suggests that it will be centred on one former patient bringing in a claim against the defendant hospital, GP, or other health provider, alleging clinical negligence by one health professional or a team. Occasionally, claims will be based on the 'direct' liability of a health provider relating to a defect in the overall organisation or the provision of resources (see Chapter 2). However, this case by case response of health providers to individual claims is being replaced by an overall strategy of risk management: assessing clinical risks and putting into place methods of managing them.

Chapter 4 demonstrates how clinical guidelines and protocols are becoming a crucial part of nursing practice. Clinical risk management emphasises teamwork, consensus and rigorous learning by experience backed by well defined record keeping in the context of laid-down treatment paths, protocols, care plans and guidelines. As well as having a role in reducing iatrogenic morbidity, active risk management also has a role in increasing the defensibility of legal claims. To defend a claim, a health provider must meet the appropriate standard of care. This does not mean avoiding all clinical accidents, but ensuring that systems and staff are in place to ensure that reasonable standards of care are met. Protocols help by demonstrating that a 'safe system', i.e. a treatment protocol based on a substantial body of expert opinion (meeting the *Bolam* standard) had been established in advance of the accident.

In GP practice, or in the field of private health care, health providers insure themselves against claims for clinical negligence. However, in the NHS hospital sector, where the biggest claims emerge, insurance is not presently available. The implications of this situation have caused concern as two factors emerged in the 1980s: an increase in overall claims and an increase in very high value claims (see section *Damages in clinical negligence* cases, above) and the fragmentation of the hospital service into individual 'stand alone' trusts. This raised the spectre that a very large claim against a relatively small trust could create a 'trust busting' crisis. As mentioned above, a claim might exceed £2 million, which would pose considerable difficulties for, say, a primary care trust with limited reserves and a turnover of less than £20 million per annum. Whilst it appears that a trust cannot become insolvent, the implications of such a 'big hit' could be to create a forced merger and, certainly, would produce a crisis diverting the trust from its primary health care task. Further, because of the internal market within the NHS, the implications of financing the payment of such a large claim might oblige the trust to increase its charges to its NHS purchasers, thus raising the prospect of driving away work to other providers and affecting the long term financial stability of the trust.

The solution to this problem has been the creation of two bodies. The Existing Liabilities Scheme (ELS) provides financial assistance for cases over £10,000 (including costs) were the clinical incident occurred before 1 April 1995. In addition, the Clinical Negligence Scheme for trusts (CNST) is a voluntary scheme enabling trusts and the remaining health authorities to pool the costs of clinical negligence, where the clinical incident occurred after 1 April 1995. The CNST will then satisfy claims, subject to an excess. Contributions would be subject to a discount if the member operates an acceptable risk management system. In this way, the trust ensures that its cash flow will not be affected by a large claim.

National Health Service Litigation Authority

The ELS and the CNST are coordinated by the National Health Service Litigation Authority (NHSLA) which operates as a legal 'back stop' to monitor proposals from trust solicitors to settle cases with the intention of ensuring best practice across the trusts, giving advice on particularly high value claims and considering the effect of 'repercussive' cases - where a decision to settle a case in the area of one trust may set off an avalanche of similar claims across the country.

Clinical Negligence Scheme for Trusts risk management standards and procedures

Risk management standards and procedures have been published in a manual of guidance issued in April 1996 by the CNST. The promotion of clinical risk management is intended to help trusts by:

1. Improving patient care.
2. Reducing claims arising out of clinical negligence.
3. As mentioned above there is an immediate incentive in potential discounts on contributions to the CNST.

Members should comply with 10 'core' standards, together with an additional standard dealing with maternity care for relevant trusts. In the first year of the scheme, members' adherence to the standards was appraised by self-assessment questionnaires. From 1996 there have been regular visits by CNST assessors. Discounts are offered subject to the score achieved.

The eleven standards established by the scheme are a useful summary of the central concerns of risk management in the clinical context:

'1. The (Trust) board has a written risk management strategy that makes its commitment to managing clinical risk explicit.
2. An executive director of the board is charged with responsibility for clinical risk management throughout the trust.
3. Responsibility for management and coordination of clinical risk is clear.
4. A clinical incident reporting system is operated in all clinical specialities and clinical support departments.
5. There is a policy for rapid follow-up of major clinical incidents.
6. An agreed system of managing complaints is in place.
7. Appropriate information is provided to patients on the risks and benefits of the proposed treatment or investigation, and the alternatives available, before a signature on a consent form is obtained.
8. A comprehensive system for the completion, use, storage, and retrieval of medical records is in place. Record-keeping standards are monitored through the clinical audit process.
9. There is an induction/orientation programme for all new clinical staff.

10. A clinical risk management system is in place.
11. In maternity units, there is a clear documented system for management and communication through the key stages of maternity care.'

Examination of a standard in detail

As time passes and information is gathered from a history of inspection visits, a comprehensive database will emerge and be disseminated to members, representing best practice.

Standard 7, which deals with consent, has as its rationale that complaints and/or litigation are less likely to be followed if patients understand to what they are consenting. Areas for assessment are:

'• Patient information is available showing the risks and or benefits of common elective treatments.
- All consent forms satisfy minimum standards and consents are obtained by a person capable of carrying out the procedure.
- Patients can obtain further information easily'

Impact on litigation

Accidents are an inevitable part of a complex clinical system but the standards set out above may reduce their impact in a number of ways. Firstly, good record keeping, allied to good communications, should prevent cases being brought simply to obtain an explanation as to why a procedure went wrong. Secondly, risk management should be used both to monitor accidents and to put in place methods of preventing them. This should prevent difficulties arising from the introduction of a new technique when it is only after a long period that anecdotal evidence suggests there is a difficulty (e.g. laparoscopic work). Thirdly, the defence of medical negligence cases can often involve a clash of medical opinion on what is the right approach. If a relevant standard is in existence and a trust has carefully thought through its standard in a particular area, for example obstetric practice, backing it with a consensus of clinical opinion and expressing it in a protocol, it is much more likely that a judge would find that this practice was acceptable as representing a reasonable and responsible body of clinical opinion.

Use of the standards in the conduct of a case

Example

A patient has elective surgery which has proved unsuccessful. The patient claims that he was not fully informed of the risks of the procedure and if he had been informed he would not have proceeded. The court applying the *Sidaway* test would ask: Did the surgeon, when obtaining consent, give the patient information on the risks of the procedure which was consistent with a reasonable body of clinical opinion? Such cases can be difficult to establish: while the patient may claim to have a vivid memory of the discussion leading to him signing the consent form the surgeon would, usually, have completely forgotten it; often the records are deficient as to what warnings were given. There may well be a dispute as to whether information given was genuinely representative of a responsible body of professional practice. An adherence to standard 7 can assist in various ways:

- The notes should refer to (perhaps, even have clipped to them) a copy of the standard leaflet telling patients of the types of risks associated with the procedure. That leaflet should be approved by the relevant clinical group and kept up to date.
- The consent form should be witnessed by a person capable of carrying out the procedure (perhaps a registrar or above) who can deal with the patient's queries and give any further information required. Crucially, such further oral information should be recorded in the notes.
- One particular problem concerns a patient who appears to understand and signs the consent form to 'please the doctor' but doesn't really follow what is going on. Nurses will be very familiar with this syndrome. Patients should be able to obtain further information, for example from a nurse or patient's advocate. Such information should be accurate and recorded

Adoption of these steps may lead to better advice and less litigation.

A nurse's 'self-defence' checklist

While many nurses will never be involved in litigation, it is important to appreciate the possibility of being involved in court action and to take measures which may assist in making defence of a nurse's practice easier.

Defence of professional practice

The *Bolam* standard suggests that practice is acceptable if a nurse can show that there is a responsible body of nursing opinion which would have taken the same approach. Keeping up to date constitutes good professional practice.

Advice and insurance

In an increasingly litigious world nurses would be wise to have adequate insurance, to join a professional association and/or a trade union to ensure that skilled legal, professional and ethical advice is available.

Good record keeping

The theme behind much of this chapter has been the importance of good record keeping in the defence of claims and practice. Nurses should pay particular attention to the guidelines on record keeping produced by the UKCC.

Clinical negligence case study

To illustrate the practical issues in clinical negligence litigation, the following case study has been created. The circumstances of the case study are serious but, fortunately, such cases are rare! *This case study is entirely fictional: any resemblance to real individuals or organisations is entirely accidental and coincidental.*

Mary Dent was a best selling author with a string of blockbuster novels to her credit. Unfortunately, her talent had a dark side: every few years her workaholic behaviour would erupt into a full blown attack of manic depressive behaviour which would involve her staying up all night, having outbursts of temper, self hurting and generally behaving intolerably to her husband and young children. After a few months she would recover. These recovery periods were generally associated with a burst of creative activity and a new novel.

Lately, she had been regularly cared for by a consultant psychiatrist at her local acute mental health trust, together with a team of psychiatric nurses. The regime established involved a care plan which was discussed and agreed by the whole clinical and nursing team. Following an acute episode she would be stabilised by drug treatment and then moved into the community to a small respite home to ease the pressure on her family. Services were provided by a resident warden (not clinically or nursing trained) and by regular visits by a community psychiatric nurse, Arthur Prefect. In view of the history of self harm, the care plan emphasised the need to ensure that any signs of agitation should be reported to the consultant with a view to returning Mary to the ward for closer observation.

Arthur, a nurse with extensive experience in community psychiatric care, had recently had a few difficulties himself. His marriage was in tatters and he had become forgetful at work. He had received a formal warning for leaving a syringe at a patient's home where it was picked up by a toddler.

One February, following an admission over Christmas, Mary moved out of the hospital and into the home. She attended the clinic once a week and received her prescription of stabilising drugs. She was visited twice weekly, as per the care plan, by Arthur, who ensured that she was taking her medication, discussed her behaviour with the warden and assessed whether the arrangement was satisfactory.

In early March, Arthur missed the first visit of the week (on a Tuesday) due to problems at home. On the second weekly visit (on a Friday) he found Mary to be much the same and, if anything, to be a little down in spirit. He felt it would be appropriate for the consultant to pay a domiciliary visit before the next clinic appointment. He planned to discuss this with the consultant at the next team meeting, on the following Monday morning. Rushing to return home to sort out a family argument he failed to make any note of the visit. On the Saturday, Mary's body was found on the local railway track where it had been hit by a train. A suicide note was left in her room.

How might these events affect Arthur? First, Mary's family are likely to bring civil proceedings alleging that lack of care led to the suicide. Second, the trust may bring disciplinary proceedings against Arthur. Third, Arthur's registration as a registered psychiatric nurse may be in jeopardy. These are considered one by one below.

Civil case of *Dent* v. *The Community Trust*

What is the legal basis of the claim?

The allegation would be that Arthur failed to come up to the standard of a reasonably competent nurse in caring for Mary and that this lack of care materially contributed to her death. She was a suicide risk and should have been better looked after. The care plan as a whole (respite home and resident warden, weekly clinic, regular medication and checks on the drug regime, together with bi-weekly nursing visits, all in the context of a team approach) was sound, but if a crucial element was missing then care fell below standard.

Who brings the claim? Who is the claim against?

The claim will be brought by Mary's husband on behalf of her estate, himself and the children. The children might be eligible for legal aid, as they have no income. Mary's husband earns too much to get legal aid (see Chapter 1). He might find that he can bring a claim under legal expenses insurance (often an 'add on' to house insurance). He might also be able to find a solicitor who would take on the case on a conditional fee basis, i.e. 'no win no fee'. (In this scheme the solicitor who fails to win the case would not charge anything but would take a 'cut' out of the damages if successful. Unless the family can afford insurance - which for this type of case is, at present, expensive - they would still have to pay the trust's costs if they lost the claim.)

In any event, this family is unusual in being able to afford to instruct the solicitor on a private basis. The claim will include the loss of Mary's life, her future loss of earnings and the replacement costs for child care. The defendant will be the trust, vicariously responsible for Arthur's acts or omissions. Arthur is not a party to the case, nor does he have his own solicitors.

Being a witness

Although Arthur is not being personally sued, he is a vital witness for the trust and would be expected to cooperate with its solicitors. They will prepare with him a witness statement that he will sign and which will be shown, with other defence statements, to the plaintiff's solicitors in exchange for their witness statements. Arthur should also see all the expert reports. In this way, well before any hearing, Arthur would clearly see the allegations made by the plaintiff's solicitor. Very few cases reach court, but were this case to do so Arthur would be expected to face cross examination. The trust's solicitors should ensure that he is fully involved and kept informed and supported.

Limitation

One common problem in litigation is the length of time it takes for many claims to be brought, often after the memories of staff have faded. A plaintiff would, normally, have 3 years to bring a claim *from the date on which the plaintiff became aware that the alleged clinical negligence caused substantial injury.* To delay beyond 3 years may prevent the patient bringing a claim (although the court does have a discretion to allow late claims). However, the date of *awareness* (knowledge) can often be years after the date of the actual negligence. Patients who suffer from brain damage (who are legally incompetent) are not caught by the limitation problem, nor are children damaged in infancy until they reach 3 years from their majority.

It follows that clinical negligence claims can be started many years after the date of the alleged negligence, making it vital that records be kept for a long period (for example, the Department of Health guidelines suggest that labour records are kept for 25 years; a claim for injury to a baby damaged at birth may have no effective limitation period as the child may be brain damaged).

Action taken by Mary's family's solicitor prior to the issue of proceedings

The first step is to obtain the clinical records. This would normally be done on a voluntary basis with the trust forwarding copies of the records on payment of their copying and administrative costs. As explained earlier (see *Pre-proceedings discovery* on p. 159) and in Chapter 7, if the records are not offered up on a voluntary basis, action can be taken to obtain them.

The expert

On receipt of the clinical records the solicitor acting for the family would instruct a nursing expert. To win the case the solicitor must show that there has been negligence *and* this negligence led to the death (if Mary would have killed herself despite the very best community care then there would be no claim). Could the principle of *res ipsa loquitur* (see Chapter 2) assist in making the claim easier by obliging the trust to show how the death could have occurred without negligence (in other words, effectively, to make the trust prove that its activity was not negligent)? This does not seem to be that type of obvious situation, such as a swab being left in, so the focus will be on Arthur's practice. Did it meet the *Bolam* standard? The nursing expert's job, based on experience, knowledge of the case and the current professional environment, will be to assess if Arthur met the standard of a reasonably competent nurse carrying out this job; if he fell below the standard, then this would support a claim for negligence. Because Arthur has experience and considerable responsibility, the expert would expect a high standard of work with the accompanying records to back up good practice. Unfortunately, in this case there is no evidence from the records that Arthur carried out the two visits, as required, in the week before the death.

In these circumstances the solicitors would send a letter before action to the trust and, if the matter could not be settled speedily, issue a case in the court.

Defendant's case

The defendant's first step is to find his own expert. The expert confirms that the care plan was satisfactory. Normally this would be a great help in defending a negligence case by demonstrating that reasonable care was taken in looking after the patient. Regrettably, here Arthur has admitted missing one visit and, whilst insisting that the second visit was made, cannot produce the records to prove it. As the warden cannot assist, then the expert suggests that the defence may be difficult. Further, the expert feels that a judge would regard Mary as a serious suicide risk and, therefore, if negligence is found the judge could well be convinced that her death was a foreseeable result of the negligence, i.e. there was causation. Further, if Mary had received better care she might well have recovered from this episode and gone on to have a productive life.

Settlement

Although the trust's solicitor would normally file a defence, faced with the risk of Arthur being disbelieved by the judge and a finding being made that Mary was left without a visit for a week, the trust decides to settle the case. However, they will not be prepared to pay the whole of the claim for two reasons: first, Arthur might be believed, and second, even if Arthur had visited and asked the consultant psychiatrists to make a domiciliary visit, Mary might have killed herself before he came. Mary's family accepts a payment of 50% of the claim, reflecting a reduction based on the possibility that the second visit is proved to the satisfaction of the judge, and the whole claim then fails.

Domestic disciplinary case and *Dent* v. *The Community Trust*

In the light of the previous warning, Arthur's nurse manager recommends to the trust that Arthur should be disciplined for failing to attend Mary on one occasion *and* failing to keep a proper record of the second visit. (Irrespective of whether Arthur visited or not on the second occasion a proper record should have been taken to assist the rest of the team and to ensure that the care plan was in place.) The domestic disciplinary proceedings, in which Arthur is represented by his professional organisation or by a trade union, might lead to dismissal. In this event Arthur might bring a claim against the trust for unfair dismissal.

UKCC proceedings

Nurses are accountable through their professional body, the UKCC (see Chapter 1). The nurse is subject to its code of conduct and disciplinary procedures. These codes are elaborated through documents setting out standards, for example for record keeping. If Arthur's act and omissions in this case could be regarded as misconduct, then it is possible that he could face removal from the register, a caution, suspension, or some other sanction.

Case study of an accident at work

Sarah Spencer works for the Goodhealth trust as a bank nurse. She has a degenerative back injury, which she declared on her application form but the trust, through an oversight, did not draw this to the attention of its occupational health department prior to her employment. Despite the odd ache and pain from her back, she is generally fit.

One late evening she was covering a geriatric ward. There were supposed to be at least two nurses on at any one time but due to staff shortages and illness Sarah was on her own. If necessary, she could call for assistance from a nearby general medical ward, but she was aware that they were short staffed.

One of the patients, an elderly, immobile, frail women was having a difficult time, unable to sleep and complaining of pain from her left hip. Sarah decided that the pain would be assisted if the patient was turned and, as the patient was quite light, she would do this without assistance. As Sarah was covering the whole of the ward she hadn't had time to read all the patients' notes and she failed to read this patient's notes, which disclosed that she was epileptic and subject to frequent fits. As Sarah handled her the patient fitted and both nurse and patient collapsed to the floor. The patient was uninjured but Sarah suffered a disabling back injury which has resulted in her having several months off work.

Finance and advice

If Sarah brings a claim how can she finance the case? She is unlikely to be eligible for legal aid, or be paying a large contribution. She may find a solicitor prepared to take her case on a conditional fee basis (see *Who brings the claim?* above); alternatively, her professional organisation or trade union may be able to assist her with immediate legal advice and long term support. All nurses are well advised to protect themselves in this way.

The legal issues

Has Sarah got a case?

The Goodhealth trust owes a duty to all its employees to take reasonable care to ensure their safety, including instituting a safe system of work (see Chapter 9). Has this duty been broken? (The duty to take care of employees - employer's liability - is often more clear cut than the duty not to be negligent in medical treatment and to prevent medical accidents. In the latter case, there can be room for more than one opinion on the correct approach. This is much more unusual in the case of accidents at work. This helps to explain why the prospects of success in a case like Sarah's are much higher than in a medical negligence case.) The trust has asked Sarah to cover a ward on her own. The ward has at least one patient who might require lifting and, if so, would need to be lifted by two members of staff. The general duty to take care is reinforced by the more specific requirements of the Manual Handling Operations Regulations 1992 (see Chapter 9). Has a management plan been drawn up to assess the patient's requirements for lifting and to train the staff in good lifting practices? If training was available, has Sarah been directed to attend? All the circumstances suggest that the trust has a case to answer.

If the trust is responsible, could Sarah have brought an action? Again, a number of factors are interwoven. Should Sarah not have worked because her degenerative back problem makes lifting dangerous? She would say that she needs to earn her living, she can do the job if suitably trained and protected, and if all nurses with back problems walked off the job there would be no one left! In any event the trust took no action on the information disclosed in her job application. Should Sarah have refused to work without more cover? Should she have checked the notes more carefully? Was this practical when she was working on her own with no one readily on call? All these factors suggest that if Sarah is successful in her case (and the odds look good), she may have to accept a reduction in her damages by virtue of her contributory negligence but her lawyer would argue that, in any event, this should be a very small amount.

Elements of the claim

Pension

Assuming that Sarah obtains a settlement or wins her case at trial, one important aspect would be that of her pension. Let us assume that Sarah had a very lengthy period off work (or indeed was never fit enough to return) she would, almost certainly, have lost some of her future pension. Whilst she works she would contribute to her pension, as would the trust. While not working, these contributions are not paid so the value of her future pension is reduced. This loss is compensated for separately from loss of earnings by a lump sum payment.

Mitigation

Sarah has gone back to work relatively quickly but what if she decided that nursing work had become too dangerous or stressful to continue? Unless her refusal to work can be supported by medical opinion that she should not be required to have mitigated her loss (see *Mitigation loss* on p. 156), she may be unable to recover loss of earnings for this period.

Provisional damages

What if Sarah's condition has stabilised before the case starts but her doctor believes that her condition is likely to deteriorate in the future, perhaps by the onset of severe osteoarthritis? If this condition is caused by the accident, rather than just being a normal organic change, it would be unfair for her not to be able to recover extra damages. Equally, it would be wrong for the trust to have to pay for a condition which might never occur. An award of provisional damages allows Sarah to apply later for more damages if a specific condition, in her case osteoathritis of the back, causes her problems in future years

Structure of the proceedings

Sarah's solicitor would conduct the case on her behalf and may seek the help of a barrister. A formal statement of her case would be filed in the court and the trust would file its own defence.

Sarah would describe what she did leading up to the accident in the form of a witness statement, which would also deal with the effect of the accident on her life. Her statement would be exchanged with statements prepared by witnesses for the trust (possibly, her manager).

Sarah would support her claim for losses by expert reports: medical reports on her current condition and prognosis, ergonomic opinion on the lifting issue and, perhaps, an employment expert discussing her employment prospects. One key area would be the production of all the relevant records, in this case the patient's records (anonomised), Sarah's employment and occupational health records, together with details of her state benefits, loss of earnings and any specific financial losses (perhaps she has had to pay for taxis, physiotherapy, etc.)

Very few accident cases reach a trial unless there is a genuine dispute on the law to be applied, an argument regarding the facts of the accident or about the amount the case is worth. Sarah seems to have a strong case so it is likely that the trust's solicitors would consider advising their client to settle once the extent of Sarah's losses are clear. They may open negotiations with Sarah's solicitor, but one very effective method is to make a payment into court. In the civil court system in the United Kingdom 'costs follow the event', i.e. the loser pays the winner's legal expenses as well as any damages. The trial is the most expensive part of an action, so the trust can put enormous pressure on Sarah by a payment into court of money in satisfaction of the whole claim. Calculation of such a 'payment in' (attractive enough to be accepted, low enough to offer the trust a discount, not so attractive that Sarah thinks the trust values the claim above the trust's estimate, etc.) combines both ruthlessness and subtlety. Failure to beat the payment in - that is, to be awarded by the Judge the same or less than the amount paid into court by the trust - means that Sarah pays both sides' costs from the date of payment in *even* if she wins the case.

In this case, Sarah would be advised to accept a reasonable 'payment in' and have her legal costs and expenses paid as well (these would be usually paid for by the trust's insurers: trusts can insure against employee and public liability claims).

Future trends

Our litigation system at present is adversarial: the plaintiff and defendant fight out their case before a judge, with experts on both sides. The process is, at present, based around the primacy of the judge and the need to ensure that judges are not left idle. The most effective way of accomplishing this is to overbook courts, so that in the event of a case settling at the last minute another one can fill the vacant slot. This produces the constant complaint of experts that they have to hold themselves ready to attend court at short notice, only to find that when they do arrive at court the case is often adjourned, or settled at the courtroom door. Cases are very expensive to bring (with legal costs often several times the damages at stake in smaller claims), which means that only the very rich or the very poor, who qualify for legal aid, can bring cases, and the complexity of claims mean that they can take years to be resolved. While personal injury - accident cases - have not suffered from the same degree of 'expertitis', they are often needlessly expensive and subject to delay.

In 1993 Lord Woolf, a senior judge, was asked by the Government to conduct a review into the problems of civil justice. In his final report, he has proposed a number of innovations which should make cases easier and cheaper to bring and simpler to resolve (HMSO, 1996). The effect of this could be to increase the number of claims brought in the future. Key aspects of the report are:

- Personal injury claims of £10,000 or under, not involving clinical negligence, should be conducted along a 'fast track' procedure, with written evidence from experts who need not attend at the trial. The use of jointly appointed single experts, or experts appointed by the court, should be encouraged. Trials should come on quickly (usually within a year) and solicitors' fees should be fixed and reduced to a proportion of the claim (Lord Woolf's initial proposal is £2500 on a claim of £10,000).
- Lord Woolf made no firm proposals in relation to smaller clinical negligence cases. He recognised that *Bolam* made it unfair to have written evidence only from experts at a trial - cross-examination of experts on the appropriate clinical standard can be vital to the appearance of fairness between both clinician and patient. He suggested that there should be pilot testing of possible methods of simplifying procedure which would still be acceptable to all sides.
- Larger personal injury cases and clinical negligence cases should be tried on the 'multi-track'. This procedure would be similar to the current procedures described in the case studies above, but the court would have much more power to step in and manage the proceedings with the aim of driving the case on to an early conclusion.
- The person bringing the case should be able to put pressure on the defendant by a method similar to 'payment in' (see above) called the 'plaintiff's offer to settle'.
- New ways of alternative dispute resolution should be encouraged, including mediation, whereby parties are brought together to resolve their differences

Nurses and crime

A nurse, like any other citizen, must obey the criminal law. Criminal liability, in broad terms, requires an *intention* to commit an offence (apart from strict liability offences, such as having a bald tyre). As this chapter has explained, it can sometimes happen that a nurse, doing his or her best and for the best of intentions, makes a mistake in professional practice. Such a mistake can involve the nurse in criminal proceedings, most probably where death results. Alternatively, a nurse can face prosecution for stealing at work, much like stealing from a supermarket, and the nurse may well have a defence, but this is unlikely to be connected with the way the nurse carries out his or her work.

The main area where nurses do risk prosecution for a criminal offence is in relation to consent for invasive procedures. As explained in Chapter 2, carrying out an invasive procedure or a physical examination on a patient without consent can constitute the crime of battery or an offence under the Offences Against the Person Act 1861. This must be differentiated from the possibility of civil liability, when the patient agrees to a procedure or examination based on inadequate information provided by the clinician. As nurses extend their role and become involved in a wider range of procedures, it is extremely important that they ensure that consents are properly obtained to avoid both criminal and civil liability.

If a nurse does face a criminal investigation it must be understood that this is a two-stage process. The police investigate the crime and submit a report to the Crown Prosecution Service, which decides whether or not to prosecute. It is absolutely vital that a nurse facing an investigation must obtain skilled professional advice at the earliest possible stage. Both the professional associations and trade unions retain lawyers to assist and, if necessary, the services of the duty solicitor scheme (which is available 24 hours a day) should be sought. What a nurse says to the police would be noted and can be used as evidence. Furthermore, silence when questioned may make it less effective at a later stage to produce an explanation which could have been offered earlier.

Litigation and expanded role

The future for nurses is an exciting one; as the next century arrives they would continue to take on an ever increasing role with enhanced technical competence, responsibility and a greater range of clinical autonomy. With this enhancement of professional responsibility would come a more central role in complaints and litigation; simply stated, if you stick your head above the parapet it is more likely that someone will try to shoot it off. Regrettable as this may be, it is now a fact of life in every profession. This suggests that nurses should put into their professional armoury not only the highest standards of technical competence but also good communication skills and a healthy respect for the law. Hopefully, this chapter has shown that with some foresight and, crucially, with good record keeping the practice of 'future nurse' can be of a high standard and eminently defensible.

References

Audit Commission (1995a) 'Setting the Records Straight: A Study of Hospital Records.' HMSO, London.

Bowles and Jones (1990) 'Medical negligence and resource allocation in the NHS.' *Social Policy and Administration*, **24**(1), 39.

Dimond, B. *Legal Aspects of Nursing*, 2nd edn. Prentice Hall, Hemel Hempstead, Chapter 2.

Emmins, C. *A Practical Approach to Criminal Procedure*, 7th edn. Blackstone, London.

The Guardian (1994) 'Trial and trial again.' 31 May.

Health Service Journal (1994) 14 April.

HMSO (1996) Access to Justice. Final Report to the Lord Chancellor on the Civil Justice System in England and Wales. HMSO, London.

Judicial Studies Board (1996) *Guidelines for the Assessment of General Damages in Personal Injury Cases*, 3rd edn. Blackstone Press, London, (i) p. 37.
Letter from NHS Management Executive to trust and health authority chief executives (1996) 1 April.
Nursing Times (1994) Pay as they sue. p. 90.
UKCC (1993) *Standards for Records and Record Keeping*. United Kingdom Central Council for Nursing, Midwifery and Health Visiting, London.

Chapter 11

Reproductive choice

Jean McHale

Today patients have an increasing range of reproductive choices. The nurse may play a direct part in guiding some of these choices, for instance the case of the teenager who approaches the nurse for advice regarding contraception, or the mother wondering whether her mentally handicapped daughter should be sterilised. In others, the nurse may not be a direct participant in the process unless a patient specifically approaches her or him for advice. Nevertheless, it is important for the nurse to be aware of the legal framework within which these choices are made and clinical procedures are undertaken. This chapter begins with an examination of the legality of the provision of contraceptive services and the question of sterilisation of the mentally incompetent adult. Secondly, we consider the regulation of the new reproductive technologies such as IVF. Thirdly, the role of the law in regulating conduct during pregnancy is explored. Finally, the legality of abortion and the involvement of the nurse in the abortion process are discussed.

Provision of contraceptive services

The nurse may be involved in providing contraceptive advice and treatment, whether as a sister in a general practice clinic or in the hospital setting. Statute states that the Secretary of State for Health has a duty to meet reasonable requirements relating to the provision of contraceptive advice/treatment of persons in England and Wales (s5(1)b National Health Service Act 1977).

While in the past the legality of undertaking sterilisation operations for contraceptive purposes was questioned, today such operations are generally accepted to be lawful (*Bravery* v. *Bravery* [1954] 3 All ER 59 at pp. 67-68.). As with any surgical procedure, before sterilisation is undertaken the patient's consent must be obtained. Consent must be obtained from the patient *himself or herself*. Her spouse/partner has no rights to participate in the consent process and may not veto the operation. The implications of the operation and the fact that there is a possibility of failure are indicated on the NHS consent form, but these should also be drawn explicitly to the patient's attention, otherwise there is the possibility that a negligence action will result. *Thake* v. *Maurice* [1986] 1 All ER 497.

One major point of controversy concerns the provision of contraceptive advice and treatment to teenagers. As seen in the section on children and confidentiality in Chapter 7, this issue came before the courts in the case of *Gillick* v. *West Norfolk and Wisbech AHA* ([1986] AC 150). If a young girl approaches a nurse seeking contraceptive advice/treatment, the nurse must assess whether the girl has sufficient maturity to appreciate the nature of the advice/treatment sought and whether she is capable of making an informed choice.

Sterilising the mentally incompetent

A mother is worried that her mentally handicapped daughter, who is in her early teens, is vulnerable to seduction. She believes that her daughter should be sterilised for her protection. She discusses her concerns with the district nurse who is helping her to care for her daughter. What should the nurse do? The mother genuinely believes that sterilisation is in her daughter's best interests. However, while the girl may have the mental age of a young child she may develop maternal feelings and in the future be capable of being a loving mother. There is also a danger in assuming that sterilisation will be a panacea when, in fact, by removing the risk of pregnancy the girl may be placed at risk of undetectable abuse. If parents and health care professionals disagree as to whether sterilisation should be undertaken then this issue should be referred to the court. The court will determine whether the proposed sterilisation operation is lawful, by assessing whether the procedure is in the girl's best interests.

Use of a 'best interests' test leaves much discretion in the hands of the courts. In *Re D*, D, an 11-year-old child from a poor background suffered from Sottas syndrome ([1976] 1 All ER 326). This condition results in accelerated growth during infancy, epilepsy, generalised clumsy appearance, behaviour problems and certain aggressive tendencies. She had reached puberty and while she had not shown any marked interest in the opposite sex, her protective mother was concerned about the consequences if she became pregnant. She wanted her daughter sterilised and her opinion was supported by her doctor.

Heilbron J. refused to authorise the sterilisation. She said that the evidence showed that there had been improvement in D's mental and physical condition. Her future prospects were unpredictable. Nevertheless, it was likely that in the future she would be able to make her own choice. Should she then realise the impact of what had happened to her, she might feel frustration and resentment. The judge emphasised that a decision to undertake sterilisation for non-therapeutic purposes on a minor was not a matter for clinical judgement alone.

In cases following *Re D* the courts have, however, shown far less hesitation before authorising sterilisation. In *Re B* ([1987] 2 WLR 1212), B was a 17-year-old woman who had a mental age of 5-6 years and was epileptic. Evidence was given to the effect that she did not understand and was unable to learn the causal connection between intercourse, pregnancy and the birth of children. However, she had the sexual inclinations of a normal 17-year-old. It was claimed that there was only a 40% chance of establishing an acceptable regime with oral contraceptives and there would be side effects. Because she suffered swings of mood and had considerable physical strength, administration of a daily dose of medication may have been impossible. B was also obese and this, coupled with the irregularity of her periods, may have made early detection of pregnancy difficult. B's mother and the local authority sought an order from the court authorising sterilisation. The court granted the order. Lord Hailsham said that the case was clearly distinguishable from *Re D*. He said:

> 'To talk of a basic right to reproduce of an individual who is not capable of knowing the causal connection between intercourse and childbirth, the nature of pregnancy and what is involved in delivery unable to form maternal instincts or to care for a child is to wholly part company with reality (p. 216).'

Lord Templeman stated that in his opinion sterilisation of a woman under 18 years should only be undertaken with the leave of the High Court. In this case it would, he said, be cruel to expose her to an unacceptable risk of pregnancy. Lord Oliver also distinguished *Re D*. He said:

> 'the right to reproduce is only valuable if accompanied by the ability to make a choice and in the instant case there is no question of the minor being able to make a choice or indeed to appreciate the desire to make one. All the evidence indicates that she will never desire a child and that reproduction will be positively harmful to her.'

The decision of the House of Lords in *Re B* has been the subject of much critical comment. For example, Lee and Morgan (1987) have asked why B was able to manage the hygienic mechanics of menstruation but not contraception, and why she was able to understand the link between pregnancy and babies but not that between sex and pregnancy. Emphasis was placed in the case upon B's mental age. But it has been suggested that this hides the complexity of the issue. For instance, a woman may have a mental age of 5 years in relation to some functions, while at the same time having far higher comprehension levels in relation to other tasks. Reference was made in *Re B* to a Canadian case *Re Eve* ([1986] DLR (4t) 1) in which the court had held that non-therapeutic sterilisation of a mentally incompetent adult was never justifiable. The House of Lords, however, disagreed and said that it was wrong to draw a distinction between therapeutic and non-therapeutic sterilisation. It is perhaps ironic in view of this that, as we shall see below, later courts appear to have drawn just such a distinction when considering whether all sterilisation operations should require judicial approval .

There are perceptible advantages in the postponement of the sterilisation decision until a mentally incompetent woman is older. Assessment of her physical and mental development may then be made on the basis of conclusive evidence, as opposed to guesswork. In B's case there was some urgency in performing the operation before she reached her eighteenth birthday because at that time the legality of treatment of the mentally incompetent adult was unclear. This issue was finally resolved 1989 by the House of Lords in *Re F* ([1990] AC 1) The House of Lords held that a mentally incompetent adult woman could be sterilised if it was in her best interests, but it stated that it would be desirable for the medical team to obtain a declaration from the court before such an operation was undertaken.

A Practice Note has been issued providing guidance as to how cases should be handled (*Practice Note: Official Solicitor: Sterilisation* [1996] 2 ELR 111). The application will be made to the High Court, patients will be represented and the Official Solicitor will attempt to ascertain the patient's views in an interview. Evidence would be required as to the patient's capacity, the risks of pregnancy, the consequences of pregnancy for the woman's health and alternatives to sterilisation. The courts have indicated that sterilisation of a mentally incompetent woman undertaken for therapeutic purposes, such as the performance of a hysterectomy upon a woman suffering from extensive menstruation, does not require judicial approval (*Re E (a minor)* [1992] 2 FLR 585). Cases involving non-therapeutic sterilisation will, however, continue to be referred to the courts. It is important to ensure that such decisions are made on the basis of the woman's best interests rather than what is convenient for the carers.

There has been a worrying trend for the courts, when authorising sterilisation, to emphasise the possibility of surgical reversal of the sterilisation operation (*Re P (minor) (wardship: sterilisation)* [1989] 1 FLR 182, [1989] Fam Law 102 and *Re M (a minor) (wardship: sterilisation)* [1988] 2 FLR 497). But as Brazier (1990) has argued, while leading experts may achieve a high level of reversals this does not mean that all clinicians can achieve this. Also, it is highly questionable whether an operation to reverse the sterilisation of a mentally handicapped person will be a priority in a financially constrained NHS.

The nurse acting as patient advocate may play an important role particularly in ensuring that in those situations in which sterilisation has not been referred to the courts, it is being undertaken for therapeutic purposes and is in that patient's best interests. An alternative approach to that presently adopted with regards to therapeutic sterilisation operations is that of at least requiring some form of second opinion to be obtained. This type of approach was favoured by the Law Commission (1995) in their report on *Mental Incapacity*. As this report now appears unlikely to be incorporated in legislation in the near future, it is important that the need for sterilisation is carefully regulated by health care professionals.

Modern reproductive technology

Developments in medical technology have, in the last half century, given much hope to the infertile. For example, a woman who is unable to conceive may receive *in vitro* fertilisation treatment IVF. This involves the egg being fertilised outside the womb and then implanted into the uterus. But use of such techniques has not been free of controversy. In response to debate generated, the Government established a committee, the Warnock committee, to examine the use of new reproductive technologies. This committee reported in 1984 (HMSO, 1984). It recommended that use of these technologies be subject to regulation. Today, modern reproductive technologies are regulated by statute in the form of the Human Fertilisation and Embryology Act 1990. This Act established the Human Fertilisation and Embryology Authority (HEFA), whose functions include the licensing of clinics providing fertility treatment (Lee and Morgan, 1991) It also grants licences for the conduct of embryo research. Not all forms of assisted conception must be licensed by the Authority. For example, artificial insemination of a woman with her partner's sperm. Not all activities may be licensed however, for example human embryos may not be placed in an animal, nor can 'cloning' – replacing the nucleus of an embryo – be undertaken (s3(3)).

There is no automatic right of access to infertility services. A woman seeking access to IVF would have to satisfy the clinic that she was a suitable case for receiving such treatment. Her eligibility is determined by reference to criteria set out in the code of practice produced by the HEFA (1995). Clinics also produce their own criteria for the approval of treatment. Criteria which would be considered include a child's need for a father, the applicants' medical histories and their commitment to bringing up children (HEFA, 1995i). That does not mean that single women would be precluded from access to infertility treatment, but the clinic would scrutinise the application and determine whether there would be any male influences in the child's upbringing. Criteria imposed by individual clinics include restrictions by reference to the age of the woman seeking treatment. Many clinics do not allow women over 35 years of age access to infertility treatment on the grounds that the success rates of treatment on older women are limited. Debates have also centred around access to IVF services for gay and lesbian couples.

Whilst there is the potential for persons denied access to IVF services to challenge this refusal in the courtroom, in practice such challenges are unlikely to be successful. For example, in *R* v. *Ethical Committee of St. Mary's Hospital, Manchester* ([1988] 1 FLR 512), R was unable to conceive. Her application to adopt a child had been rejected because of her criminal record relating to prostitution and brothel keeping. She sought IVF treatment. A consultant at the IVF clinic rejected her application. This decision was supported by the hospital's infertility ethical committee. (Bodies undertaking infertility treatment must establish ethical committees to which problematic decisions relating to access to such treatments may be referred.) Schiemann J. said that the committee was in essence an informal body. If the committee in a particular case refused to give advice to a consultant or did not come to a majority view on a decision, he didn't see that the court could compel it, either to give advice or to enter into a particular investigation. Schiemann J. did not rule out the possibility of judicial review:

> 'If the committee had advised, for instance, that the IVF unit should in principal refuse treatment to anyone who was a...jew or coloured, then I think that the court might well grant a declaration that that was illegal.'

But he stressed that the committee was a talking shop for professionals and a court should be cautious before intervening. It appears that such challenges are unlikely to be successful in the future unless they are manifestly unreasonable/indefensible. This was illustrated in the later case of *ex parte Seale* (1994 unreported). S, a 36-year-old woman, was denied IVF treatment. It was said that there was a need to ration resources and treatment was generally less effective in those women who were over 35 years of age. The court was not prepared to overrule the clinic's decision to refuse her treatment on the basis that it was irrational.

The code of practice issued by the Human Fertilisation and Embryology Authority provides that couples contemplating use of modern reproductive technologies should be given counselling as to the implications of undertaking such therapy (HEFA, 1995). The nurse may be involved in such counselling.

A nurse may object to her participation in the use of certain techniques such as IVF which involve gamete or embryo manipulation on religious or cultural grounds. Section 38 of the 1990 Act gives nurses and other health professionals the right to refuse to participate in such treatments by expressing a conscientious objection to participation.

Surrogacy

A surrogate is the term used to describe a woman who carries the child of another. This practice has been undertaken for centuries. Recently, however, surrogacy been linked with modern reproductive technologies. It is argued that surrogacy can be both a necessary and helpful method of alleviating infertility. It may assist women who have suffered repeated miscarriages and might be appropriate in a situation in which a women was medically unable to cope with the trauma of pregnancy although she was capable of caring for a child once born. In practice, it appears that surrogacy is regarded as appropriate only in exceptional cases. The British Medical Association (BMA, 1990) has recommended that surrogacy:

> 'should only be considered as a last resort where the commissioning couple suffers from infertility due to a medically recognised disorder and where all appropriate means for enabling them to have a child have been tried and failed.'

There are reasons why surrogacy is seen as problematic. Firstly, there may be conflicts between the natural mother and the commissioning parents with the surrogate seeking to keep the child. Secondly, much discussion around surrogacy has concerned the commercialisation of the practice. It has been argued that making money out of the surrogate process is ethically unacceptable. The Warnock Committee was opposed to the commercialisation of surrogacy. The Surrogacy Arrangements Act 1985 provides that it is an offence to arrange a commercial surrogacy agreement (s2(1)) or to advertise surrogacy services (s3). No prosecutions have as yet been brought under the Act. The legislation is targeted at surrogate agencies. The commissioning mother and the surrogate do not commit an offence under this statute (s2(2)). Whilst the law does not ban surrogacy agreements, they are however *unenforceable*. For instance, if a surrogate decided to keep the child, the commissioning parents could not demand that the child was handed over by her (s36(i) Human Fertilisation and Embryology Act 1990).

Regulating the conduct of the mother during pregnancy

Nurses and midwives have long played an important role during pregnancy and in childbirth. Today midwives are involved not only in the delivery itself but through ante-natal classes in the process of health education regarding birth. While over time the guidance and advice given to pregnant women has increased, few active constraints are imposed during pregnancy. While there is an active debate in the USA as to the extent to which women should be constrained by law during pregnancy, attempts to use the law to regulate behaviour in the period prior to birth in this country have been unsuccessful (Robertson, 1995). This is illustrated by the case of *Re F (in utero)* ([1988] 2 All ER 193). The court was faced with the issue of whether a fetus could be made a ward of court. F's mother had led a nomadic existence around Europe. She had disappeared and those caring for her were concerned that the fetus in her womb would suffer harm if the woman did not seek medical attention. The court, however, refused to make the child a ward of court, stating the court's jurisdiction under wardship did not extend to an unborn child.

It seems unlikely that at present English law will be used to compel behaviour during pregnancy (although contrast the attitude of the law regarding childbirth itself, below). Were such compulsion to be sanctioned, this would require radical revaluation of the role of the nurse and midwife in caring for the mother.

Freedom to choose where to give birth

During the last century the birth process has become increasingly medically dominated. Much use is made of technological interventions in pregnancy. Today only around 1% of women give birth in their own homes. There are a number of reasons why this is the case. It may be regarded as 'safer' for the mother. Hospital births may be more convenient for the hospital team. Some suggest that the increase in surgical interventions during pregnancy is motivated by fear of a 'malpractice crisis' with doctors increasingly prepared to advise patients to undertake caesarean sections to avoid the risk of litigation should the pregnancy prove problematic. Indeed, the need for the number of caesarean sections presently undertaken has been questioned. In some instances a caesarean section may be the only alternative otherwise mother, child, or both may be at risk of death. A child may be in the breech position and if the child's head becomes stuck, brain damage may result. At the same time there are risks attached to the performance of a caesarean section. Evidence has been given to the effect that for example, the operation may put a woman at a 6 to 11 times increased chance of death during childbirth or haemorrhage. In addition, if the woman becomes pregnant again, the risk of rupture to the scar on the uterus may mean that another caesarean operation will be required (Anderson and Strong, 1988).

There is some evidence of a shift in policy regarding the conduct of childbirth. A report issued by a House of Commons Committee stated that 'the policy of encouraging all women to give birth in hospital cannot be justified on grounds of safety' (House of Commons Health Committee Session 1991-92 Maternity Services). A government committee chaired by Lady Cumberlege published a report in 1993 called *Changing Childbirth: Report of the Expert Maternity Group*. The report identified three key principles. The woman should be the focus of maternity care provision. Maternity services should be readily and easily accessible to all, and services must be effective and efficient. The NHSME has recommended that statements for implementing these recommendations should be included in contracts between purchasers and providers (EL(94)(9) NHSME).

Today, the law regulates childbirth in two specific ways: first, by statute in the form of the Nurses, Midwives and Health Visitors Act 1997 and second, through common law interventions regarding enforced caesarean sections.

A midwife or doctor must attend the birth

The woman's preference regarding her choice of birth is subject to her being able to obtain a doctor and nurse who are willing to deliver a child at home, a choice which may ultimately depend upon whether she is prepared to or indeed able to pay for an independent midwife to attend her. It is a criminal offence under s16 of the Nurses, Midwives and Health Visitors Act 1997 for a person other than a registered midwife or registered medical practitioner to attend a woman in childbirth. This provision is aimed at protecting the mother and ensures she has expert care to hand when she needs it. There is an exception for sudden and urgent necessities, as where a midwife is summoned, but before she arrives the mother gives birth, with the assistance of her partner. Student midwifes are allowed to attend a mother in childbirth as part of their training, but they must be supervised by a qualified practitioner (s16(2)(b) Nurses, Midwives and Health Visitors Act 1997). The practitioner supervising the midwife remains accountable for the conduct of the birth.

The mother may object to the presence of a midwife/doctor when she gives birth. In such a situation, the midwife should inform the mother of the legal position and that she risks prosecution should she refuse to give her consent.

Birth plans and compelling a caesarean section

Today it is common for women to agree with their midwife a plan for the conduct of their birth. This states such matters as whether a woman would receive pain relief, etc. But what if in a particular situation a midwife believes that it is necessary for the health of the woman to depart from the birth plan? Treating in the face of a previously stated refusal may, as we saw earlier, render the midwife or doctor liable in the tort of battery (see Chapter 5). However, in some situations this may not prove practical. A woman states her wishes as regards a natural 'low tech' birth, but then complications develop; should the birth plan be followed? It could be argued that it should not if all the possible eventualities have not been foreseen. Any birth plan which is drawn up should be undertaken only after the implications of refusal of certain types of treatment, and the problems if an emergency arises have been pointed out to the woman. Where it is proposed to go ahead in the absence of express consent then, wherever possible, a court order should be sought.

Take a situation in which it is discovered late in pregnancy that a caesarean section is required. The woman says that she is a Jehovah's Witness, she is opposed to blood transfusions being given and does not want a caesarean section. What if the consequence of the patient's refusal of a medical procedure such as a caesarean is that both woman and fetus will die? Such a problem came before the English courts in the 1992 case of *Re S* ([1992] 4 All ER 671). S was 6 days overdue giving birth. The health care team wanted to undertake a caesarean section because, as the fetus was in transverse lie, any attempt at a normal birth carried a very grave risk of rupture to the uterus. S, who was a Born Again Christian, refused the operation. This was because it would have involved a blood transfusion, which was against her religious beliefs. The hospital sought a declaration from the court, which was granted by Sir Stephen Brown. The decision – notable for its brevity – has been criticised (Grubb, 1993). In his judgment, Sir Stephen Brown made reference to a United States case *Re AC* ([1990] 573 A.2d 1235 at 1240), in which a court had been prepared to authorise a caesarean section on a pregnant woman. But, while courts in the United States have been prepared to order enforced treatment upon pregnant women, *Re AC* is far from a clear authority supporting the use of enforced caesareans. On appeal in that case, after the death of the woman on whom the caesarean had been ordered, the court stated that the operation should not have been authorised. Grubb has suggested that the only plausible basis for the decision is the right to refuse treatment being outweighed by the interests of society in preserving life where there is potential for survival. But, as he comments, if this is the basis for the decision it goes beyond anything to have been decided previously. The decision to authorise treatment in the face of the patient's refusal in *Re S* may have been regarded as exceptional, indeed the Royal College of Obstetricians and Gynaecologists, in a consultation paper published in 1994 stated, 'It is inappropriate and unlikely to be helpful or necessary to invoke judicial intervention to overrule an informed and competent woman's refusal of a proposed medical treatment, even though her refusal might place her life and that of her fetus at risk.' (RCOG, 1994) Nevertheless, recently the courts have indicated that they are prepared to authorise enforced caesareans. In *Tameside* v. *Glossop* ([1996] 1 FCR 753), a declaration was made by the court to the effect that a pregnant woman suffering from schizophrenia, sectioned under the Mental Health Act 1983, could undergo procedures consequent upon birth, including a caesarean section if required, as this constituted necessary treatment under section 63 of the 1983 Act. In addition, in subsequent cases *Rochdale NHS Trust* v. *Chowdury* (1996); *Norfolk and Norwich NHS Trust* v. *W* ([1996] 2 FLR 613) reported in the press in September 1996, the courts have authorised caesarean sections in situations in which a woman had previously indicated her objection to such procedures (Hewson, 1996). This issue now requires urgent re-evaluation. It appears that a number of women who allege that caesarean section operations were performed upon them without their consent are about to bring legal proceedings.

No English court has yet been faced with the question of whether to authorise treatment on the basis that the patient who is refusing care has a dependent family. The issue has arisen in the United States, where the courts have been prepared to uphold the right of the patient to refuse treatment regardless of the impact upon the patient's family (*Norwood Hospital* v. *Munoz* [1991] 564 NE 2d 1017). It is submitted that this is the correct approach to take and that, whatever the consequences, if a competent patient makes a clear refusal of treatment that refusal should be respected.

There is a further point. While a woman is liable to prosecution should she refuse the assistance of a midwife, there are no explicit statutory powers enabling a woman to be compelled to be taken from her home and brought to hospital for treatment other than, for example, those which relate to treatment of the mentally ill, and it is unlikely that the court would sanction such a procedure at present.

Postnatal care

The nurse or health visitor may be involved in providing antenatal care to mother and baby. What if the nurse believes that a mother s/he is attending is abusing drugs and that the home is unsuitable? In this situation, the nurse should bring the matter to the attention of the social services. They may decide to take action and, if necessary, use one of the orders available to them under the Children Act 1989 (for fuller discussion see Chapter 6).

Liability for injuries in relation to conception and childbirth

Negligence of health professionals, whether in providing advice regarding sterilisation or during the conduct of childbirth, may lead to litigation. The process of childbirth is fraught with difficulties and mistakes are easily made. In the debates on the existence of a malpractice crisis in health care (see Chapter 10), obstetrics and gynaecology are frequently cited as examples. The general principles of negligence are discussed in Chapter 2. Here a few specific points are considered briefly.

Where a child is born handicapped as a result of conduct which it is claimed is negligent, then a claim may be brought against a nurse or doctor. The Congenital Disabilities (Civil Liability) Act 1976 allows an action to be brought by a child who has suffered a disability (s1(3)). This Act was passed following the debate and legal action which arose from the use of the drug thalidomide. This drug had been given to pregnant women to counteract morning sickness, and it was alleged that as a consequence children had been born handicapped. An action can only be brought under the 1976 Act if the child is born alive and has lived at least 48 hours (s4(2)). It must be shown that the disability which the child has suffered was the result of an occurrence which affected the mother/father's ability to have a child, or affected the mother during pregnancy or affected mother or child during birth. Situations in which an action may be taken include a child being born handicapped due to negligence during the birth. To bring a claim under the Act, it must be shown that the nurse or midwife owed the mother a duty of care (s4(2)). Any damages awarded under the Act may be reduced if the parents were contributorily negligent in the harm caused.

In practice, it seems that liability is difficult to establish, with few claims having been brought. Many of these claims will fall on the grounds that the negligence itself did not cause the harm suffered. It is perhaps of interest in view of the earlier discussion as to the obligation of the pregnant woman towards her fetus that an action may not be brought by a child against her mother for negligent conduct under the 1976 Act. The one exception to this is in a situation in which the fetus is injured by negligence of the mother when driving a car and the mother knew or ought reasonably to have known that she was pregnant (s2 Congenital Disabilities (Civil Liability) Act 1976).

An action at common law cannot be brought on behalf of the child on the basis that the injuries the child suffered were such that s/he would be better off never having been born. The Court of Appeal rejected such a 'wrongful life' claim in the case of *McKay* v. *Essex Area Health Authority* ([1982] 2 All ER 771), on the basis that the court could not assess the award of damages satisfactorily to assess the difference between never having been born and a life of disability. In addition, it was argued that to allow such damages here could encourage health care professionals to advise on an abortion, rather than risk subsequent litigation where a child was born handicapped. Parents can, however, bring claims for the cost of bringing up a severely disabled infant born due to medical negligence during pregnancy or childbirth. The possibility of such litigation illustrates the importance of risk management and following protocols where available (see Chapter 10).

Abortion

Background to the existing law

Abortion is one of the most controversial of all clinical procedures (Dworkin, 1993; Keown, 1988). It was made a criminal offence in England by the Offences Against the Person Act 1861 s58 and s59. In addition, the Infant Life Preservation Act 1933 made it an offence to destroy the life of a child capable of being born alive. This remained the position until 1967, subject to a limited exception being recognised for abortions undertaken to preserve the life of the mother or to ensure that she was not rendered a 'physical and mental wreck' (*R* v. *Bourne* [1939] 1 KB 687). In 1967, after much heated debate the Abortion Act was passed, largely through the efforts of the Liberal MP David Steel. This legislation was amended in 1990 by clauses inserted into the 1967 Act by the Human Fertilisation and Embryology Act 1990. The introduction of abortion legislation was accompanied by a heated ethical debate. On the one hand the use of abortion was strongly advocated by those who supported a 'pro-choice' approach. Abortion was, however, opposed by those who can be loosely grouped under the heading 'pro-life' and who regarded the abortion process as that of the killing of a human person or potential person (Dworkin, 1993). The legislation, as can be seen below, has provided no absolute rights to any of the parties to the abortion process. There is no right to abortion on demand, the father has no rights, and nor has the fetus. In many respects the abortion decision can be viewed as one characterised by medical determination and domination.

The nurse should be broadly aware of the law as it relates to abortion, and particularly the Abortion Act 1967 for a number of reasons. Acting in her or his role as patient advocate, the nurse may be involved in counselling and advising a woman who is contemplating an abortion. Also, the nurse may have fundamental religious objections to abortion. When can s/he legitimately refuse to participate?

When is an abortion lawful?

An abortion is lawful if authorised by two registered medical practitioners who are of the opinion, held in good faith, that one of four grounds laid down in the Abortion Act 1967 has been met.

Social abortions

First, an abortion is allowed if the woman is less than 24 weeks pregnant and continuation of the pregnancy would involve a risk, greater than if the pregnancy were terminated, of injury to her physical or mental health or that of any child in her family (s1(1)a). This category – the so called 'social ground' – is the provision under which most abortions are authorised. It leaves considerable room for the exercise of medical discretion. For example, there is controversy as to whether the psychological pressure placed upon women in certain cultural groups to have a male child provides sufficient justification for the abortion of a female fetus. 'Social' abortions can only be undertaken in the first 24 weeks of pregnancy, but the Act does not state from when this time runs. There are a number of possibilities (Murphy, 1991), such as the date of the woman's last period, date of implantation or date of fertilisation

Other grounds for abortion

The other grounds for abortion under the 1967 Act are not subject to an express time limit. An abortion may be undertaken if termination of pregnancy is necessary to prevent grave permanent injury to the physical or mental health of the pregnant woman (s1(1)b). An abortion is also lawful if continuation of the pregnancy involves a risk to the life of the pregnant woman greater than if the pregnancy were terminated (s1(1)c). Finally, an abortion may be undertaken if there was a substantial risk that if pregnancy were to continue the child would be born seriously handicapped (s1(1)d). The statute does not define 'seriously handicapped'. It is unclear whether this refers to a handicap which the child would be born with if the pregnancy continues, or if it extends to conditions such as Huntington's chorea, which will not develop until a person is around 40 or 50 years old (Morgan, 1990).

Emergency abortions

The Act states that an abortion must be authorised by two medical practitioners (s1(1)). However, one doctor may authorise an abortion if it is the only way of averting an immediate risk to the woman's life or grave permanent injury to her (s1(4)).

No right to an abortion

It must be stressed that there is no right to abortion on demand. The ultimate decision regarding the performance of an abortion is a matter of clinical judgement after discussion between the doctor and the patient. Just as a woman has no right to demand an abortion, neither does her husband/partner have any legal right to be consulted or to veto the abortion decision (*Paton* v. *Trustees of the British Pregnancy Advisory Service* [1978] 2 All ER 987; C v. *S [1988] QB 135).* Also, English law does not recognise the fetus as possessing legal rights (*Paton* v. *British Pregnancy Advisory Service*).

Selective reduction

The development of IVF treatment led to a difficulty relating to abortion. In the course of IVF treatment, in order to increase the chance of a successful implantation, more than one embryo is usually transferred into the womb. In some situations, this may result in a number of embryos becoming implanted. Such a multiple pregnancy may constitute a serious risk to the mother's health. The amendments made to the Abortion Act 1967 in 1990 included a provision to the effect that it was lawful to remove one or more embryos as long as one of the grounds for abortion under the 1967 Act had been met (s5(2)). These provisions do not only apply to multiple pregnancies arising as a result of infertility treatment. There was recent controversy regarding a press report that a consultant had performed selective reduction on a woman with twins who sought an abortion under the 'social' grounds of the legislation (*The Guardian*, 1996).

Abortion and the incompetent patient

While a competent adult patient can clearly consent to an abortion, difficulties may arise if it is proposed to undertake an abortion upon a teenager or a mentally incompetent woman. A teenager may be competent to consent herself if she is regarded as of sufficient maturity under the test in *Gillick* (see Chapter 6). But what if she refuses an abortion? While in theory the parental power of consent may override the refusal of a competent child, if a teenager wanted to keep her baby then any dispute between her and her parents should be immediately referred to the court. It would, it is suggested, be unlikely that the court would force a girl to undergo an abortion.

While it may be seen as good practice to seek court approval before an abortion is performed on a mentally incompetent woman there is, strictly speaking, no need for such an order to be made before the abortion goes ahead (*Re SG* [1991] 6 BMLR 95 (Fam Div)). The decision to undertake an abortion upon a mentally incompetent adult must be reached on the basis of what are her best interests. The nurse as patient advocate may play an important role in ensuring that the patient's interests are properly taken into account in making this decision.

The Law Commission (1995i) in its report on Mental Incapacity, expressed concern that abortions were being undertaken on young women with learning disabilities without proper investigation into their ability to consent, and best interests. It suggested that, before an abortion is performed upon a mentally incompetent woman, there should be a requirement for a certificate to be obtained from an independent medical practitioner that the abortion is in the woman's best interests.

Where should the abortion be carried out?

Section 1(3) of the Act provides that abortions must be undertaken in an NHS hospital or in a place which has been approved by the Secretary of State for the purposes of undertaking abortions. This provision created difficulties in relation to the abortion pill, the drug RU486. It was intended that this would be administered to patients at GPs' surgeries. To cover this section 1(3)(a) was enacted which provides that:

> 'The power under subsection (3) of this section to approve a place includes a power in relation to treatment consisting primarily in the use of such medicines as may be specified in the approval and carried out in such manner as may be so specified, to approve a class of places.'

This power has not yet been exercised, thus at present RU486 may be lawfully administered to patients only in hospital. Even if a GP's surgery is approved as a relevant place, this only covers the initial administration of the drug. The patient is then usually discharged. At this time the drug is still acting. Surely each patient's home cannot be included in any designation! These problems require urgent consideration by Parliament.

Role of the nurse in prostaglandin abortions

While the 1967 Act provides that the pregnancy must be terminated by a registered medical practitioner the nurse plays a major role in certain abortion procedures. In prostaglandin abortions, the doctor inserts a catheter into the womb via the cervix in order to create a space between the womb and the amniotic sac containing the fetus. This may cause abortion. If not, various other steps are undertaken, such as attaching a catheter to a pump propelling prostaglandin into the womb. These are mostly carried out by a nurse or midwife. However, the legislation made no reference to the nurse, simply referring to the doctor's role in the process. The Royal College of Nursing went to court to obtain an order to clarify the legality of the nurse's involvement in the abortion process (*RCN* v. *DHSS* [1981] AC 800). The House of Lords held that the doctor need not do everything with his own hands. Lord Diplock stated that

Parliament had contemplated that, as with other hospital treatment, abortion would take place as a team effort: junior doctors, paramedics, nurses and other members of the health care team would each undertake those tasks which would be, in accordance with a responsible body of medical practice, entrusted to a member of staff possessed of their respective skills. The involvement of the nurse in the process was lawful.

Conscientious objection

Abortion is an exceedingly sensitive ethical issue on which many people hold very strong beliefs. The 1967 Act itself takes account of this. Section 4 of the 1967 Act provides that:

> 'no person shall be under any duty whether by contract or by any statutory or other legal requirement, to participate in any treatment authorised by this Act to which he has a conscientious objection: Provided that in any legal proceedings the burden of proof of conscientious objection shall rest on the person claiming to rely on it...'

The section does, however, go on to provide that:

> 'Nothing in subsection (1) of this section shall affect any duty to participate in treatment which is necessary to save the life or to prevent grave permanent injury to the physical or mental health of a pregnant woman.'

Thus, a nurse who is a devout Roman Catholic may refuse to participate in an abortion procedure save in an exceptional situation, such as where a woman is brought in bleeding profusely from the uterus and it is clear that without an abortion she will die.

While the Act gives the nurse the right to refuse to be involved in clinical procedures, the statutory right of conscientious objection does not extend to those persons more remotely connected to the abortion process. In *Jannaway* v. *Salford AHA* ([1988] 3 All ER 1079) a secretary who was a Roman Catholic refused to type a letter referring a pregnant woman to a consultant with a view to securing an abortion. Ultimately she was dismissed. She claimed that the dismissal was unfair and that the conscientious objection provision under section 4 protected her. Her claim was rejected in the House of Lords. Lord Keith said that 'participation' for the purposes of section 4 meant actual participation in the treatment administered in a hospital or other approved place.

Liability if the 1967 Act is not complied with

There has been some discussion as to whether the procedure set out in the 1967 Act has to be complied with before for example an intra-uterine device is inserted after intercourse or before the 'morning after pill' is given. In some situations, failure to comply with the Abortion Act 1967 may result in a criminal prosecution. Section 58 of the Offences Against the Person Act 1861 states that it is an offence to use an instrument with the intention of procuring a miscarriage. What constitutes 'carriage' for these purposes is somewhat unclear (Montgomery, 1997) but advice has been given by the Department of Health that post-coital contraception should only be administered in a period of 72 hours after conception.

Today, abortion may also be undertaken through administration of the drug RU486. This drug is clearly abortifacient since it operates after the ovum has become implanted. It is almost certain that it must be given in accordance with the 1967 Act.

Failure to comply with the 1967 Act may also place those performing the abortion at risk of prosecution under the Infant Life Preservation Act 1929 for the offence of child destruction. Section 1(1) of this Act provides that:

> 'Any person who with intent to destroy the life of a child capable of being born alive by any wilful act causes the child to die before it has a life independent of its mother shall be guilty of the offence of child destruction and shall be liable on conviction to life imprisonment.
>
> But that no person shall be found guilty under this section unless it is proved that the act which caused the death of the child was not done in good faith for the purpose only of preserving the life of the mother.'

No offence will be committed under this Act as long as the provisions of the Abortion Act 1967 have been complied with. Were a prosecution to be brought under this section, a court would have to consider whether the fetus was 'capable of being born alive'. Some guidance as to what this term means has been given in the case of *C* v. *S* ([1988] QB 135). Here, the court rejected the claim that a fetus of 18–21 weeks was 'capable of being born alive'. Lord Donaldson said that while at 18–21 weeks the cardiac muscle is contracting and primitive circulation is developing – and therefore the fetus could be said to be developing real and discernible signs of life, nevertheless it was unable to breathe either naturally or with the aid of a ventilator.

The mature fetus

If a hysterectomy is undertaken in the later stages of pregnancy, the fetus may be born alive. An infant who has taken breath and shown signs of life after being expelled from the womb is entitled to a full birth certificate and to be fed and cared for. If a nurse leaves the infant to die then a prosecution for murder or manslaughter may result. For example, in *R* v. *Hamilton* (*The Times*, 16 September 1983), an infant was discovered after abortion to be 33 weeks rather than 23 weeks old. The infant – clearly alive after delivery – was left in the sluice room for some 15 minutes before being transferred to the intensive care unit. The infant survived. Dr Hamilton was charged with attempted murder although, ultimately, the magistrates decided that there was no case to answer. The nurse as patient advocate should be concerned to safeguard the rights of the infant patient. If the nurse finds that a baby has been born and is at risk of death, s/he must immediately take steps to secure the infant's survival. The nurse should also report the condition in which the infant was found and any perceived deficiencies in care.

There is a greater chance that the fetus will be born alive in a situation in which an abortion is undertaken late in pregnancy. One reason why abortion may be undertaken late in pregnancy is because of delay in the initial referral. Clarke quotes a Royal College of Gynaecologists' study which found that 20.5% of women who had abortions between 20 and 23 weeks had been referred at 12 weeks but had then experienced delay in obtaining a consultation and appointment for treatment (Clarke, 1987). As far as possible, any delay from the initial point at which a woman sees her doctor to any abortion should be minimised.

Registration of births and stillbirths

When a woman gives birth, whether to a living infant or to a stillbirth, then the doctor or the midwife who has attended the woman is under a statutory duty to inform the responsible medical officer of that fact (s124 NHS Act 1977; Notification of Births and Deaths Regulations 1982; SI 1982 No 286). A stillbirth is the term used to describe a child born dead after 24 weeks of pregnancy and which did not breathe or show any sign of life (s41 Births and Deaths Registration Act 1953, as amended by the Still Birth Definition Act 1992).

The Births and Deaths Registration Act 1953 requires the mother or father to inform the Registrar of a birth within 42 days (s2). If either of them is unable to do so, then there is a duty upon the occupier of the house, any person present at the birth or any person who has charge of that child to give the Registrar that information (s2(1)(2)). A midwife may be such a person. If the birth has not been registered within 42 days then the Registrar can compel any qualified informant to come before him to provide information and to sign the Register, having first given them 7 days' notice in writing. Where a stillbirth is being registered, the informant must provide the Registrar with a certificate stating that the child was not born alive. This certificate should have been signed by a registered medical practitioner or by a certified midwife who was present during the birth or who subsequently examined the dead body. A birth is classified as a stillbirth where the foetus is more than 24 weeks old. (StillBirth (Definition) Act 1992).

References

Anderson, G. and Strong, C. (1988) 'The premature breech; caesarean section or trial of labour.' *Journal of Medical Ethics*, **18**, 18.

Brazier, M. (1990) 'Sterilisation: down the slippery slope.' *Professional Negligence*, **6**, 25.

British Medical Association (1990) *Surrogacy: Ethical Considerations; Report of a Working Party on Human Infertility Services*. BMA, London.

Clarke, L. (1987) 'Abortion – a rights issue.' In *Birthrights* (eds R. Lee and D. Morgan). Routledge, London.
Cumberledge, Lady (1993) *Changing Childbirth: Report of the Expert Maternity Group.* DOH, London.
Douglas, G. (1991) *Law, Fertility and Reproduction. Modern Legal Studies.* Sweet and Maxwell, London, p. 195.
Dworkin, R. (1993) *Life's Dominion: An Argument About Euthanasia and Abortion.* Harper Collins, London.
Grubb, A. (1993) 'Treatment without consent: Adult.' *Medical Law Review*, 931.
The Guardian (1996) 'No new issue' in abortion of twin.' 5 August.
Hewson, B. (1996) 'Women's rights and legal wrongs.' 146 *NLJ*, 1385.
HEFA (1995) *Code of Practice.* Human Fertilisation and Embryology Authority, (i) para 3.18(a).
Keown, J. (1988) *Abortion, Doctors and the Law.* Cambridge University Press, Cambridge.
Law Commission (1995) *Mental Incapacity*, Report No. 231, HMSO, London, (i) para 6.10.
Lee, R. and Morgan, D. (1991) *The Human Fertilisation and Embryology Act 1990.* Blackstone Press, London.
Lee, R. and Morgan, D. (eds) (1987) 'A lesser sacrifice: sterilisation and the mentally handicapped woman.' In *Birthrights.* Routledge, London.
Montgomery, J. *Health Care Law.* OUP, Oxford, p. 362.
Morgan, D. (1990) 'Abortion – the Unexamined Ground.' *Crim LR* 687.
Murphy, J. (1991) 'Cosmetics, eugenics and ambivalence; the revision of the Abortion Act 1967.' *Journal of Social Welfare and Family Law*, 375.
Report of the Committee of Inquiry into Human Fertilisation and Embryology 1984 HMSO (Warnock Committee Report). Cmnd 9314.
Robertson, J. (1995) *Children of Choice.* Princeton University Press, Princeton.
Royal College of Obstetricians and Gynaecologists (1994) *A Consideration of the Law and Ethics in Relation to Court-authorised Obstetric Intervention.* RCOG, London.

Chapter 12

The end of life

Jean McHale

The nurse frequently plays an important role in caring for patients at the end of life whether, for instance, in the area of palliative care and the hospice movement, or in the intensive care unit. Many difficult issues arise at the end of life. A patient who is terminally ill and who is in considerable pain may tell the nurse that he wants to die. What should the nurse do? A mother is presented by the midwife with a child who is grossly handicapped and screams for the child to be taken away from her. How far is the medical team required to keep that child alive? A young man is killed in a road accident, and the nurse is approached for advice by the man's father as to whether his son's organs could be used for transplantation. While the nurse may be the primary carer and required to take primary responsibility at the end of life, in many situations s/he will be acting as part of a treatment team. This area also gives rise to a number of difficult issues for the nurse as patient advocate.

This chapter considers a number of important legal questions at the end of life. It begins by examining the approach taken in English law to issues of active and passive termination of life. There is much discussion as to whether there is a right to die. As will be seen, there is only a right in the sense that a patient can choose to end his or her own life – English law does not sanction active euthanasia, though in certain situations withdrawal of treatment is lawful. The second section considers the definition of death. In the final section the legal regulation of organ donation is examined and some proposals considered for law reform.

Ending life – criminal liability

A seriously ill patient may plead with a nurse to 'put him out of his misery'. However grave his agony, if the nurse complies s/he may be prosecuted for murder. English law does not recognise active euthanasia. In *R* v. *Carr (Sunday Times*, 30 November 1986). Dr Carr had injected a massive does of phenobarbitones into a patient with inoperable lung cancer. The judge, Mars J., emphasised that every patient was entitled to every hour that God had given him, however seriously ill that patient might be. The jury eventually acquitted Dr Carr.

However, in 1992 Dr Cox was prosecuted and convicted of attempted murder (*The Times*, 22 September 1992). (He was not charged with murder because at the time of the investigation the body of the alleged victim had been cremated and thus the exact cause of death could not be established.) Dr Cox had been treating a 70-year-old woman terminally ill with rheumatoid arthritis and also suffering from gastric ulcers, gangrene and pressure sores. She expressed a wish to die. When repeated doses of heroin did not ease her agony, Dr Cox gave her a dose of potassium chloride – a poison. Dr Cox was convicted and sentenced to 1 year's imprisonment suspended for 12 months.

In *R* v. *Arthur* (*The Times*, 5 November 1981) the non-treatment of an infant resulted in a criminal prosecution. A baby, John Pearson, was born with Down's syndrome but apparently suffering no other complications. Dr Arthur, a paediatrician caring for the child, wrote in the notes, 'Parents do not wish it to survive, nursing care only', and he prescribed a strong pain killing drug DF118 – a drug not normally given to infants. The baby died a few hours later. Dr Arthur was charged with murder but this was later reduced to a charge of attempted murder. While he was eventually acquitted. The case left open many difficult issues as to what care a child must be given and whether the health care professional could cease treatment if it is believed that further care is hopeless. The judge in *R* v. *Arthur* described the doctor's conduct as being a 'holding operation'. However, it has been suggested that the administration of the drug DF118 – an appetite suppressant – amounted to a positive act. This case must now be considered in the light of the *Bland* decision where the court indicated that a decision to cease life-sustaining treatment will not necessarily give rise to criminal liability (see below).

Generally, there will only be liability in criminal law where a nurse or doctor has undertaken a positive action. The law does not usually impose liability for omissions. Nonetheless, as will be seen below, there may on occasions be only a narrow line between these two categories.

If a nurse discovers that a doctor has deliberately ended the life of a patient, what should the nurse do? In two cases in which doctors were prosecuted for allegedly ending the life of the patient, the prosecutions followed action taken by the nursing staff. Dr Arthur was prosecuted after a report was made by a nurse who was a member of a pro-life organisation. Dr Cox's prosecution followed a report made by a nurse, Sister Hart, regarding his conduct. She stated that she was required by the UKCC code to speak out – relying on clauses 2 and 11. The nurse may be subject to disciplinary proceedings if she fails to report such an incident (Fletcher et al., 1995).

What should a nurse do if, as in the case of Sister Hart, she knows that the patient's life has been ended but that the patient has expressed a wish to die? Does the duty which the nurse owes to the patient mean that s/he should take into account the fact that this patient had expressed a wish to die? While the nurse is obliged to act in the patient's interests, it must be the case that the nurse should be prepared to report what is a serious breach of criminal law.

The law places parents under particular obligations in relation to the care of their children and holds them accountable, not only for their actions but also for their omissions. If parents, perhaps motivated by some personal ethical belief, fail to seek medical care for a gravely ill child and as a result the child dies, they may be prosecuted under s1 of the Children and Young Persons Act 1933 which makes it an offence to neglect the care of the child. A prosecution may also be brought for murder or manslaughter. In *R* v. *Senior* ([1899] 1 QB 283), the parents were members of a religious sect which objected to the use of medical assistance and medicines. Their child fell ill but they did not seek medical help. The child died of diarrhoea and pneumonia. Evidence was given to the effect that had the child received medical treatment then she would probably have lived. Although no medical care had been given, the child had been generally well treated. It was held that the parents' actions amounted to neglect under s1 of the Prevention of Cruelty to Children Act 1896 – the statutory predecessor to the 1933 Act which provided that:

> 'If any person...who has the custody, charge or care of a child...wilfully neglects...such child in a manner likely to cause such child injury to its health that person shall be guilty of a misdemeanour.'

In this case the parents were found guilty of manslaughter because their actions had caused or accelerated the child's death. But, more recently, the courts have held that neglect by itself will not necessarily mean that a prosecution for manslaughter will succeed (*R* v. *Lowe* [1973] QB 70). However, in 1993, parents who believed in homeopathic remedies and who failed to seek conventional medical help for their child, who subsequently died, were convicted of manslaughter (*The Independent*, 29 October 1993).

Administration of pain-killing drugs

The nurse charged with ending the life of a suffering patient cannot plead that this was a 'mercy killing'. No such defence is recognised in English law. But, in some situations, administration of strong pain killing drugs is justifiable even though repeated doses will, over time, have the effect of cutting short the patient's life. In *R* v. *Bodkin Adams*, Dr Bodkin Adams was prosecuted for murder ([1957] *Crim Law Review* 365). Dr Adams had cared for many elderly patients and had been a beneficiary in the wills of a number of those patients. One 81-year-old widow who had suffered a stroke was prescribed heroin and morphia by Dr Adams and later died. Dr Adams was named as a beneficiary under her will. At the trial the judge, Devlin J., said that there was no special defence of mercy killing. But a doctor was entitled to do all that was proper and necessary to relieve his patient's suffering even if the measures used had the effect of incidentally shortening that patient's life. Brazier (1992) has stated that:

> 'This analysis introduces into the law the double-effect principle much debated in philosophical circles, whereby if an act has one of two inevitable consequences, one good and one evil the act may be morally acceptable in certain circumstances.'

The doctrine of double effect has been used in the context of abortion. The approach taken in *R* v. *Bodkin Adams* has been questioned. The UKCC (HL, 1994) has commented that:

> 'to prohibit euthanasia...yet permit the use of narcotics to alleviate pain even at doses which will dramatically shorten life or even bring it to a close within a very short period, is no longer a sustainable position.'

Reg Pyne, former assistant registrar of the UKCC, suggested that nurses generally saw the doctrine of double effect as hypocritical (HL 21-4, 1994). The first duty of the nurse and other health care professionals is to care for the patient. A decision to administer strong pain killing drugs is not to be taken lightly. However, if that decision is made and the incidental effect is that a patient's lifespan is reduced then, at present in English law, that will not amount to murder.

Suicide

While euthanasia is unlawful a patient may take his or her own life. Suicide has not been a crime in this country since the Suicide Act 1961 came into force. As noted in Chapter 5, a patient may refuse life-saving treatment, and indeed to treat a patient who has refused such treatment without his or her consent may lead to an action in the tort of battery and possibly to a criminal prosecution. But if the patient asks a nurse to bring some lethal drug and to sit with him or her while s/he dies, the nurse must not do so. Section 2(1) of the Suicide Act 1961 provides that assisting suicide is an offence. To establish a prosecution it must be shown that the defendant knew that the person was intending to commit suicide, assented to this and encouraged them in their attempt (*AG* v. *Able* [1984] 1 All ER 277).

Should euthanasia be legalised?

As with abortion, euthanasia is an exceedingly emotive subject (Dworkin, 1993). It has been argued that recognition of active voluntary euthanasia is simply a logical extension of the right to commit suicide, and that it is part of giving respect to the autonomy of the individual. Furthermore, it has been suggested that the present position, which sanctions the withdrawal of treatment while at the same time rejecting active euthanasia, is inconsistent and illogical.

A number of attempts have been made over the years to legalise euthanasia in this country. Nevertheless, some strong voices have been raised in dissent. One fear is that of the 'slippery slope'. It is argued that it is easy to 'slip' from recognition of voluntary active euthanasia to involuntary euthanasia undertaken without an individual's consent, for convenience or other purposes. Critics of euthanasia point to the experience in the Netherlands. In that country, while euthanasia itself is unlawful, legislation provides that prosecutions will not be brought against doctors who terminate the lives of their patients as long as they comply with certain procedures. Claims have been made that procedures have not been complied with and that abuses have occurred (Keown, 1991).

The 'slippery slope' argument was one factor which influenced the Select Committee of the House of Lords to reject the introduction of euthanasia legislation in this country (HL, 1994). A further difficulty is, who would administer euthanasia? Should it be the same persons who normally care for patients? Were it to be introduced it would have considerable implications for the role of the nurse. Recognition of active termination of life is opposed by those who see the function of health care as one of 'curing', not killing. While the euthanasia debate seems set to continue, any alteration of the law to sanction active euthanasia appears unlikely in this country, at least in the near future.

Withdrawing treatment

While a health professional may not end a patient's life with a positive action, in some situations it is lawful to withdraw treatment in a hopeless case. This section considers the well known case of Tony Bland and the situations in which treatment may legitimately be withdrawn. It should be noted here that 'withdrawal' includes not only the decision to, for instance, remove a feeding tube, but also the decision not to administer a particular treatment should a relapse take place.

The Bland case

In the case of *Airedale NHS Trust* v. *Bland* ([1993] AC 879), Tony Bland was injured at the disaster at the Hillsborough football ground in 1989. His chest was severely crushed and as a result he suffered hypoxic brain damage. He entered a persistent vegetative state (PVS). He was fed through a nasogastric tube. After several years, during which he showed no noticeable sign of improvement, an application was made for a court order allowing the withdrawal of treatment. The order was granted. The judges in the House of Lords emphasised the fact that English law did not authorise euthanasia; however, there were situations in which there was no longer a duty to continue all treatment. The court recognised that there was a distinction in law between actions and omissions, and that usually failing to act was not culpable in criminal law. The House of Lords classed withdrawal of tube feeding where continued treatment was no longer in that patient's best interest as being an omission, not an act. In a case such as *Bland*, continued treatment was of no benefit to him as there was no prospect of his condition improving. What amounted to the patient's 'best interests' was to be assessed by reference to a responsible body of professional practice, the *Bolam* test (see Chapter 2). While obtaining a court order is a civil procedure, in practice a successful murder prosecution involving medical staff who remove an artificial feeding tube after a court order has been obtained is highly unlikely. Indeed, an attempt to bring a prosecution after the death of Tony Bland was unsuccessful (*R* v. *Bingley Magistrates Court ex parte Morrow* 13 April 1994, unreported).

The *Bland* case does not simply recognise that there may be a point at which it is legitimate to discontinue treatment and remove artificial feeding. It was suggested in the House of Lords that in some situations there may be a *duty* to do so. Lord Browne Wilkinson held:

> 'If there comes a stage where the responsible doctor comes to the reasonable conclusion (which accords with the views of a responsible body of professional medical opinion) that further continuation of a life support system is in the best interests of the patient, he can no longer lawfully continue that life support system, to do so would constitute the crime of battery and the tort of trespass to the person.'

The exact scope of this duty is yet to be determined. It should be noted that it may be in the patient's best interests to discontinue treatment even though the relatives believe that treatment should be continued (*Re G* [1995] 2 FCR 46). One emotive question which remains to be answered after *Bland* is whether spoon feeding will be classed along with feeding through a nasogastric tube as medical treatment .

Unauthorised termination of treatment

While a health care professional may be authorised to remove a patient from life support systems, that does not mean that any person switching off such a machine will be held to have simply omitted to act. If a mother comes into the ward and turns off the life support system because she believes that her son has suffered enough, and has not obtained a court order, she may be prosecuted for murder.

Applying Bland

In *Bland* the diagnosis was clear. The relatives and health care professionals were in agreement. Nevertheless, the House of Lords noted that this was an exceptional case and that subsequent cases should be referred to the courts. In a number of later cases, withdrawal of treatment has been authorised but difficulties remain. In *Frenchay* v. *S* ([1994] 2 ALL ER 403), S had taken an overdose and suffered consequent brain damage. The consultant caring for him said that S was in a persistent vegetative state and had no chance of recovery. S was being fed through a gastronomy tube in the stomach wall. This tube became dislodged. The question was, should it be reinserted? The parents were divided as to whether treatment should be continued, while the health care professionals caring for S were opposed to the continuation of treatment. On appeal, the Court of Appeal upheld the decision of the judge at first instance, supporting withdrawal of further treatment. The case of *Frenchay* differs from that of *Bland* in certain respects. In *Frenchay* there was no question of removing the feeding tube, as it had already become dislodged. In *Bland*, great emphasis was placed upon the fact that the patient was in an irreversible condition. One controversial aspect of *Frenchay* is that it was suggested that the diagnosis of PVS was by no means conclusive. In addition, the court in *Bland* had stated that there should be clear evidence as to the patient's medical condition, preferably from two doctors. Here, because the tube had become dislodged, the urgency of the case led to evidence being given by only one doctor. The *Frenchay* case may not be an isolated one. It is likely that many of these decisions concerning treatment withdrawal may arise in similar emergencies. This may be particularly problematic, since recent research has questioned the efficacy of diagnosis of PVS in many cases (Andrews et al., 1996). It appears that a considerable number of patients have, in the past, been the subject of misdiagnosis. A Practice Note which provides guidance as to conduct of cases concerning withdrawal of treatment states that a patient should be in PVS for a period of more than 12 months before diagnosis is made (Practice Note (Vegetative State) [1996] 2 FLR 375).

In *Bland* it was suggested that whether a patient had fallen into a hopeless condition was to be assessed by reference to the *Bolam* test - the view of a responsible body of professional practice. But in *Frenchay*, Sir Thomas Bingham MR indicated that the courts would be prepared to review the doctor's assessment as to what was in the patient's best interests. This is a different approach, which may involve considering factors such as the quality of life the patient would enjoy were treatment to be continued. It appeared to be a shift away from *Bland* in that the court is undertaking the task of determining what amounts to 'best interests' rather than leaving this as a matter of judgement by health professionals (Kennedy and Grubb, 1994).

Very difficult decisions concern withdrawal of treatment in a situation in which the patient is not in a PVS but is gravely handicapped and incompetent. Prior to *Bland*, a number of cases came before the courts concerning the decision to withhold treatment from handicapped children. If a child is born suffering from a serious handicap and after counselling the parents say they cannot cope and they do not want treatment to be continued, what can be done? This may be a situation in which it is sought to withdraw treatment. Such decisions are not to be taken lightly. Counselling should be given as to the nature of the handicap, prognosis and future survival rates. Handicaps can vary dramatically, from the Down's Syndrome baby with a duodenal atresia where a simple operation to remove the complication can ensure that the child survives well into the thirties, to the anencephalic infant born without upper hemispheres of the brain whose survival rate is likely to be no more than a few weeks.

Where there is doubt as to whether treatment should be continued, it is advisable for an application to be made to the court to approve a course of non-active treatment. If such an order has been obtained then any subsequent criminal prosecution, if death results, would be unlikely. The court makes an order as to future treatment on the basis of what is in the child's best interests. At first sight this may be regarded as similar to the *Bland* type case. But there are differences. In *Bland*, the situation was hopeless with no prospect of recovery in the case of an adult unconscious patient. Ascertaining 'best interests' in the case of individuals who are incapacitated because of grave handicap may be more difficult. The court may be in effect assessing what is and what is not an adequate quality of life.

In *Re B* ([1981] 1 WLR 1421) a baby was born with Down's syndrome and a duodenal atresia. The parents did not want her to have an operation to correct the atresia. They believed that it would be better for her to die within the next few days. The hospital, however, informed the local authority. B was made a ward of court. The issue of whether to continue treatment was left to the court to determine. At first, the court authorised the operation. However, later B was removed to a different hospital where differences arose as to whether treatment should be given and this led to the matter being referred back to the court. The Court of Appeal authorised the operation. Lord Justice Templeman said:

> 'There may be cases I know not, of severe proved damage where the future is so certain and the prognosis so uncertain and where the life of the child is so bound to be full of pain and suffering that the court might be drawn to a different conclusion, but in the present case the choice which lies before the court is this whether to allow an operation to take place which may result in the child living for 20 or 30 years as a mongoloid or whether (and I think that this must be brutally the result) to terminate the life of a mongoloid child because she also has an intestinal complaint.'

The court decided that the operation should go ahead, as once B had the operation she was perfectly capable of living a full life to the normal Down's syndrome lifespan. In a number of subsequent cases, the courts have shown themselves willing to approve an order not to pursue active treatment. These cases extend beyond the very young infant to include children of some 3 or 4 months old. In *Re C* ([1989] 2 All ER 782), the Court of Appeal approved an order in respect of an infant born prematurely, suffering from severe hydrocephalus with severe mental and physical handicaps. She was not gaining weight and the medical prognosis was that her condition was hopeless. On appeal, while the court approved the decision to cease active treatment, it said that the following words (in the original order of the judge):

> 'The hospital authority be at liberty to treat the minor to allow her life to come to an end peacefully and with dignity...'

should be deleted because of the risk that misunderstanding would be caused by the phrase 'allow her life to come to an end'.

The meaning of 'best interests' was explored further in the case of *Re J* ([1990] 3 All ER 930). J was born nearly 13 weeks premature weighing only 1.1 kg. At birth, J was put on a ventilator and though later taken off the ventilator he suffered relapses and had to be reventilated. He was seriously brain damaged and appeared also to be blind and deaf. In addition, it was likely that he would be totally paralysed. An application was made for an order to the effect that if J again suffered a collapse he should not be ventilated. The Court of Appeal made the order. Lord Donaldson MR, referring to a Canadian case, suggested that in deciding whether to withdraw treatment:

> 'the court must decide what the patient would choose if he was able to make a sound judgement.'

This child endured a very poor quality of life. He had already been ventilated for very long periods and had an exceedingly unfavourable prognosis. In reaching his decision, Lord Donaldson emphasised the fact that mechanical ventilation was an invasive procedure which would cause the child distress.

Lord Donaldson's approach has been criticised. As Wells et al. (1990) comments, it is artificial to use a subjective test in relation to neonates and young children because there is no way of knowing what they would have wanted. Much uncertainty, however, remains in this area.

The nurse may play an important role in ensuring that any decision to withdraw treatment is carefully made. Any decision reached must be on the basis of the best interests of the child, as opposed to what may be convenient for parents or for health care professionals. If the nurse believes that a child is not being given suitable care, this must be reported to the appropriate authorities.

Withdrawal of ventilator support

The question still arises whether it would be possible to withdraw a patient from a ventilator if that patient has not been declared brain stem dead. Health care professionals would need to assess whether withdrawal from the ventilator can be said to be in the patient's best interests. In 1996 the court authorised the withdrawal of ventilator support from an infant brain damaged by meningitis. The girl was blind, deaf and unable to respond to her parents (*ReC(a baby)* [1996] FLR 43).

Reforming the law

After the *Bland* and *Cox* cases, a Select Committee of the House of Lords was appointed to consider the issue of euthanasia and withdrawal of life-saving treatment (HL, 1994i). They suggested that 'treatment limiting decisions' of incompetent patients should be taken by all those involved in the patient's care and the patient's close relatives. If there was no agreement as to what care to pursue, then the issue could be referred to a new forum. The basis for withdrawing treatment should be that 'treatment may be judged inappropriate if it will add nothing to the patient's wellbeing as a person'. The Law Commission recommended that discontinuation of artificial sustenance to an unconscious patient who has no activity in the cerebral cortex and no prospect of recovery should require either court approval (consent of an attorney or manager) or, if allowed by an order of the Secretary of State, a certificate by an independent medical practitioner (draft Bill clause 10(2)). They were uneasy as to the use of 'best interests' as the test to apply in making the decision to withdraw treatment. This was because, while it could be said not to be in the patient's best interests to continue treatment, it could be argued that it is not in the patient's best interests to end the treatment. Nevertheless, they went on to recommend that the factors in the 'best interests' checklist should be considered when making this decision (see Chapter 5).

With respect, this appears to be in effect performing some kind of mental gymnastics. Their proposal that approval may be given by one of three possible decision-makers also creates difficulties. Surely there are different policy reasons for leaving this decision to a court than there are for leaving it to a medical practitioner? If these proposals are introduced as legislation, then clearer guidance is needed for the health care professional. In this area, legislative reform appears unlikely in the immediate future. Difficult balancing issues remain. Decisions of treatment withdrawal would need careful re-evaluation in the light of medical evidence.

Living wills

A patient is involved in a motorway crash and is brought unconscious into hospital. It appears that there are serious physical injuries and it is likely that should the patient recover, he will be paralysed and severely brain damaged. The relatives say that the patient has made a living will, and that this states that in such a condition the patient would not have wanted to have treatment continued. What should be done?

A living will is a statement made by the patient before s/he becomes incapable of making his or her own decision, to the effect that should the patient became incapacitated what treatments s/he would not want pursued. Judicial acceptance has been given to advance refusals of treatment (*Re T* [1992] 4 All ER 649). One common form of such advance refusal is the card carried by the Jehovah's Witness. A living will is in some respects an extension from such a card. However, although a living will may provide a useful guide as to what treatment should or should not be given it is important to note that such a document may not authorise an action which is currently unlawful, for example euthanasia. In addition, a patient cannot use a living will to require the health care team to continue all possible treatments regardless of expense and efficacy. The UKCC (1996i) has noted that:

> 'Although not necessarily legally binding, they can provide very useful information about the wishes of a patient or client who is now unable to make a decision and should therefore be respected.'

At present there is no legislation governing living wills and many uncertainties remain regarding their application. The courts may accept them in principle but it has been suggested that a number of safeguards are required to ensure that the living will properly reflects the patient's wishes. The Law Commission (1995i) recommends that there should be a rebuttable presumption that living wills are valid if in writing, signed by the maker and witnessed. However, the Law Commission does not believe that a patient should have the right to refuse all treatment. It suggests that a patient should not be able to refuse 'basic care', by which is meant care to ensure basic bodily cleanliness and direct oral hydration and nutrition (Law Commission, 1995ii). The BMA in its document *Advance Statements About Medical Treatment*, also believes that a person should not be able to refuse basic care. Death of a patient refusing such 'basic' care may be particularly unpleasant for the nurses caring for that patient and for the other patients on the ward. Yet at the same time, a patient who is competent can decide to die slowly by refusing all food. Should a patient not be allowed to make a similar decision through a living will?

A further difficulty with the living will is that a person's view may change over time – what may seem a totally intolerable state of health at 20 years of age may not be regarded as intolerable at all at 75. Lapse of time between the will being initially drawn up, and then later interpreted, needs to be taken into consideration when applying the will. Another issue is the applicability of a living will to a woman who later, when the issue of treatment and the validity of the living will arises, is pregnant. It has been suggested that before a living will is made, women of childbearing age are asked to consider the possibility of becoming pregnant (Law Commission, 1995 iii, para 5.24).

Drafting living wills – the role of the nurse

If living wills become commonly used the nurse may be involved in advising the patient as to how a living will should be drawn up and the implications of such living will. The BMA (1995ii) has stated that 'Hospital managers and GP practice managers need to consider how to respond to the increasing desire of patients to plan ahead on the basis of accurate health information and advice.' The BMA notes that some hospitals have specialist counsellors who provide support and information and that home visits are provided. It states that 'Hospice outreach services and community nurses may also become involved in carrying out such a role' (BMA, 1995iii). This is in contrast with an earlier statement by the RCN to the effect that the nurse should not be involved in drawing up living wills (RCN, 1992). It is submitted that the RCN approach is preferable. If a patient wishes to draw up a living will, s/he should be able to seek advice for that purpose, but it should come from outside the clinical team. It is important to ensure that any decision is perceived to be wholly independent of any considerations of convenience in resource allocation.

Continuing powers of attorney

In some situations although a living will may exist, it may not help the health professional. It may be insufficiently specific, it may have been made a number of years ago and doubts may be raised as to the extent to which this now reflects an individual's interests. One alternative is for a person to be appointed to make treatment decisions on behalf of the mentally incompetent person. Such a person is known as a 'treatment attorney'. At present while a person can appoint another person to make decisions about his or her financial affairs, if s/he becomes incompetent, this does not apply to treatment (Enduring Powers of Attorney Act 1985). The Law Commission (1995(iv)) has suggested that the law should recognise such attorneys and allow patients to nominate a person to act in their best interests when they themselves become incapable of making a decision. They do, however, comment that the power of any such attorney should be limited and, for example, would exclude the power to authorise the removal of 'basic care' (draft Bill clauses 16(3)(c) and 9(8)). But recognition of proxy decision making may bring its own problems. Not least is the fact that ascertaining a person's wishes may be difficult if it is a long time since they have exercised the power of appointment (BMA, 1995). Nevertheless, it may at least assist in providing some guidance regarding an exceedingly difficult issue.

'Do not resuscitate' orders

Hospital nurses will be familiar with the practice of placing a 'do not resuscitate' (DNR) order in the patient's notes. But on what basis should this decision be made? A joint BMA/RCN report considered the use of DNR orders (BMA/RCN, 1993). They recommended that use of a DNR order may be considered if it is believed that cardiopulmonary resuscitation is unlikely to succeed, or if it is contrary to the patient's express wishes, or if a patient is resuscitated s/he would be unlikely to have a quality of life which s/he would find acceptable. In ascertaining quality of life, the guidelines suggest that as far as possible the patient's views should be obtained, but if this is impossible then the patient's close relatives should be consulted. The guidelines leave the ultimate decision whether to make a DNR order in the hands of the consultant although they do state that patient involvement in these decisions is 'valuable' and 'important'. While discussion is not mandatory, they suggest that careful enquiry should be made of those patients who are thought to be at risk and the results of these discussions should be included in the hospital notes.

But does this go far enough to safeguard the patient's interests? There is a danger that a patient is only involved in the process to ensure his/her compliance with the decision. While the guidelines recommend that consultations about DNR orders should be made with members of the clinical team, the ultimate responsibility for the decision is placed in the hands of the consultant. S/he has the task of assessing an individual patient's quality of life. However, as Schutz (1994) commented:

> 'this is a highly subjective process which requires a depth of relationship that consultants are unlikely to achieve. Even though the consultant has legal responsibility for the patient's treatment in relation to resuscitation there needs to be more emphasis on the team approach.'

Once a DNR order has been made the guidelines suggest that all members of the health care team should be informed and that the order itself should be subject to a regular review. The nurse may play an important role in monitoring the operation of DNR orders in her capacity as patient advocate.

The use of a DNR order has now been given judicial approval in principle in the case of *Re R* ([1996] 2 FLR 99). In this case, the court upheld a DNR order in relation to a 23-year-old man who had cerebral palsy, brain malformation and learning difficulties and while not in PVS was in what was termed a 'low awareness state'. Evidence was given that he was physically and neurologically deteriorating. The consultant treating R was of the view that it was in R's best interests to allow nature to take its course the next time he had a life threatening incident. The judge made an order stating that it would be lawful to withhold the administration of antibiotics in the event of the patient suffering a life-threatening infection and to withhold cardiac pulmonary resuscitation. The DNR order here was drawn up in line with the RCN/DOH guidance.

At present, DNR orders have a comparatively low public profile and many persons are unaware that such practices are used. In view of this it is suggested that it should not be left to informal guidance. Other countries, such as the USA, have legislation governing DNR orders. While until now legislation on this matter has been rejected in this country, were legislation to be introduced governing living wills, it is submitted that statutory criteria for the use of DNR orders should be introduced.

Death

When are health care professionals entitled to hold that a patient is dead? There is no statutory definition of death in English law. However, for many years clinical practice has recognised brain stem death as the point at which death occurs (Royal College of Physicians, 1996). This has now been confirmed by the courts. In *Re A* ([1992] 3 Med Law R 303) the court held that a child who was being supported on a ventilator, and who had been declared brain stem dead, was dead for all intents and purposes and thus a doctor who had disconnected the ventilator was not acting unlawfully. This approach was supported by the House of Lords in *Bland*. In that case their lordships confirmed that those patients in a state of 'cognitive death' with irreversible damage to the upper hemispheres of the brain and who were in a persistent vegetative state were not legally dead.

Certification of death must be undertaken by a doctor (Births and Deaths Registration Act 1953 s22). It is not the role of the nurse to undertake this task. Certain deaths must be notified to the coroner by the doctor who is certifying death. These include death related to suspicious circumstances.

Organ transplants

Transplant technology has developed considerably over the past few decades. A wide variety of transplants of organs and tissues is increasingly undertaken, ranging from kidneys and bone marrow to heart and lungs. The nurse frequently plays an important part in the transplant process. The nurse may work as a transplant coordinator. S/he may counsel patients who are considering whether to undergo a transplant. S/he may also have to attend the patient's body after the removal of organs in the haemodialysis unit or intensive therapy unit. In this part of the chapter the regulation of transplantation is considered.

Cadaver transplants

A patient has been injured in a car crash and dies later in hospital. It is hoped that the patient's organs can be used for transplantation into a patient urgently awaiting a donor, but can they be lawfully used?

The current law regulating cadaver transplants is contained in the Human Tissue Act 1961. Removal of the organs must be authorised by the person who is 'lawfully in possession of the body' (s1(1) Human Tissue Act 1961). If death has taken place in hospital, this is usually the hospital authorities (s1(7)). The organs may be removed if the deceased person had agreed to the use of his or her organs, whether in writing through, for example, the use of a donor card or orally in the presence of two witnesses during his last illness. This will lead to transplants being authorised *unless* there is reason to believe that the deceased withdrew his request.

If there is no donor card the organs may still be used if this is authorised by the person lawfully in possession of the body. S/he must show that s/he has no reason to believe after making such inquiries as are reasonably practical, that the deceased has expressed an objection to the body being used for transplants and that the surviving spouse/relative of the deceased does not object to transplantation (s1(2)). The Act requires enquiries to be made of spouse/relative only (s1(2)). This does not take into account the fact that a person may be estranged from relatives and may be in a long term relationship outside marriage. The legislation does not define what amounts to 'reasonable enquiries'. It has been suggested that it would be reasonable simply to enquire of the spouse or close relative as to whether they or another person has expressed an objection (Skegg, 1984). It is an open question whether, if the organs are needed sufficiently urgently, it would be justifiable to remove them without making any enquiries of the relatives. Despite the technical legal uncertainty surrounding this point, in practice it appears that organs will not be removed unless the donor's relatives have been consulted.

The actual transplant must be undertaken by a doctor who has satisfied him/herself that two sets of brain stem death tests have been performed and have proved negative. Eyes may be removed by a doctor who has ascertained that life is extinct or by a person acting on the instructions of a doctor (s4(a) Corneal Tissue Act 1986). The doctor must be satisfied that the person in question is sufficiently qualified/trained to perform completely the removal. The qualified person must be either satisfied life is extinct by examination or be satisfied on basis of statement to that effect by a doctor.

If it appears that an inquest may have to be held on a body or a post mortem will be required, then organs may not be removed without the coroner's consent (s1(5)). The difficulty with this is that in referring the matter to the coroner, the delay may render the organs useless. The Home Secretary has issued a circular regulating this issue. It is stated that the coroner's consent should be refused only where there may be later criminal proceedings in which the organ might be required as evidence, or if the organ is/might be the cause/partial cause of death or if its removal might impede further investigations.

Commercial dealing in organs

In the late 1980s there was a major scandal when it was discovered that individuals were being offered money to come to this country from Turkey and sell their organs for transplantation. This led to disciplinary proceedings being brought against a number of doctors, with one being struck off the General Medical Council's register. One result of the scandal was the passage of the Human Organ Transplants Act 1989 which made it a criminal offence to pay persons to donate organs or to undertake any other commercial dealing in organs from live donors or from cadavers (s2).

Live organ donations

If it is sought to use living persons as organ donors then first, the appropriate consent must be given and second, certain statutory provisions in the form of the Human Organ Transplants Act 1989 must be complied with. It appears generally accepted that organ transplantation from adults is the type of operation which may be lawfully undertaken (Brazier, 1992i). Nonetheless, it is doubtful whether a competent adult is capable of lawfully consenting to the removal of a vital organ with death as a consequence, if nothing else because such removal would lead to the surgeon being prosecuted for murder.

In addition, doubts have also been expressed as to the legality of transplantation of animal organs to humans because of the risk to the intended donor (Mason, 1990). At present such transplants are not being undertaken on humans but this is now the subject of review by a new body, the Xenotransplantation Interim Regulatory Body (Fox and McHale, 1997).

In some instances it may be sought to use a child as a donor. Although child patients are frequently bone marrow donors, use of child patients as solid organ donors is infrequent and it appears that surgeons are unwilling to use child patients as donors. In the Court of Appeal in *Re W (a minor)* ([1992] 3 WLR 758), Lord Donaldson said that the statutory right of children over 16 years to consent to treatment contained in the Family Law Reform Act 1969 did not apply to organ donation. Whether a child is able to consent to his or her organs being donated would have to be decided using the common law. Here, the only guidance available is the *Gillick* test that a child can consent to a procedure if s/he has sufficient maturity to consent to that procedure. In the case of a very young child, parental consent would be required. In practice if donation is sought from a child patient, of whatever age, parental consent should be obtained. One particular difficulty may be in ensuring that consent is freely given, bearing in mind the very highly charged emotional situation in which such a decision would be made. If it is sought to use a mentally incompetent adult for a donor then the matter should be referred to the court who will consider whether such a procedure could be said to be in the patient's best interests (*Re Y* [1996] 2 FLR 791).

Human Organ Transplants Act 1989

Transplants between related donors

A further repercussion of the Turkish organ scandal was that the Human Organ Transplants Act 1989 placed a number of limitations upon the practice of live organ donation. It is now an offence for a person living in the UK to remove an organ intended to be transplanted into another person or to transplant an organ from one living person to another living person unless the criteria set out in the Act are followed. If the donor intends to give an organ to a relative, it must be shown that the person into whom the organ is to be transplanted falls within a prescribed group. This group is drawn very broadly to include not only parents and children but extends to, for example, uncles and aunts of the half blood (s2(2)). The genetic relationship is established by a genetic fingerprinting test (Human Organ Transplants (Establishment of Relationship) Regulations 1989 SI (1989 No. 2107) and it is an offence to remove organs unless such a test has been undertaken.

Transplants between unrelated donors

While the legislation does allow transplants between unrelated donors, various limitations are placed on such donations (s2(6)). These reflect the concern of the legislators to protect potential donors from exploitation. Transplants between unrelated donors are governed by the Unrelated Live Transplant Regulatory Authority (s2). The Authority must be satisfied that the donor has received no unauthorised payments. The donor must be given and must understand an explanation of the medical procedures for, and the risks involved in, the removal of the organ. This consent must be given freely without coercion/offer of an inducement. The donor must understand that s/he is entitled to withdraw consent but has not done so. Both donor and recipient must be interviewed by a person who appears to the Authority to be suitably qualified to conduct such interviews. This person must make a report to the Authority as to whether the criteria for donation have been satisfied.

Reforming the system?

There is a grave shortage of organs and long transplant waiting lists. For example, in 1992 there were 4343 patients waiting for a kidney transplant but only 1622 transplants were undertaken. Many proposals have been made for reform of the present system (New et al., 1994). These extend from clarification of the provisions of the Human Tissue Act 1961 to legislation allowing automatic removal of organs from the deceased save where the person had made an indication to the contrary before death. Below are considered briefly some of the main suggestions for reform.

One option is the introduction of opting out legislation (New et al., 1994). It allows organs to be removed without express permission being obtained, unless a deceased person had expressed an objection before his or her death. There is some evidence that the introduction of such a scheme in countries such as Belgium has increased the supply of available organs. Nevertheless, proposals to introduce opting-out legislation into this country have met opposition. There are fears that persons may feel pressurised into not opting out. Opposition to such legislation may come from certain religious/cultural groups who are unhappy with transplantation or who do not accept brain stem death. Opting out may also lead to relatives' wishes being ignored. In practice, however, in countries where opting out legislation has been introduced, the donor's relatives are still consulted. This raises the question as to whether the introduction of opting out legislation would lead to a radical increase in supply. A number of unsuccessful attempts have been made to introduce opting out legislation into this country; nevertheless, at present it appears questionable whether this will be undertaken.

Another alternative is that of required request. This practice is much used in the United States. There, hospitals are obliged to set up procedures enabling routine enquiries to be made of patients and their relatives as to whether organs may be used if the patient subsequently dies. Required request does not appear to have led to any dramatic increase in the number of organs available for harvest in the USA. This may be due, at least in part, to the fact that there have been practical problems with the operation of required request in the USA, not least the fact that in many hospitals the procedures have been badly established and operated. It has, however, been argued that required request can impose considerable burdens on hospital staff in having to make time-consuming enquiries of potential donors and relatives.

In the absence of legislative change there have been attempts to increase the supply of organs by improving the present system. For many years, members of the public have been encouraged to carry donor cards indicating their willingness to donate organs, although there has been some scepticism regarding the effectiveness of such a scheme (New et al., 1994). A computerised organ donor register was introduced in 1994, the NHS Organ Donor Register, which allows individuals to have their wishes regarding organ donation entered on to computer. Transplant coordinators can contact the Organ Donor Register as a means of identifying the donor's wishes. Intending donors may tick a box on their driving licence application form expressing their wish to donate organs and this information will be entered onto the Organ Donor Register.

One method of facilitating the supply of organs for transplantation which provoked considerable controversy is a practice known as 'elective ventilation' (McHale, 1995). Patients with an intracranial haemorrhage, in a hopeless condition and who were regarded as suitable donors, were transferred to intensive care units where they were ventilated to facilitate use of their organs for transplantation. This procedure was controversial in that when the patient is transferred to the intensive care unit s/he may not have been declared brain stem dead. This practice was halted because it was stated to be illegal. While medical procedures can be performed upon a mentally incompetent patient if in their best interests, the extent to which this is applicable in relation to the mentally incompetent patient is uncertain. Elective ventilation is not undertaken for the patient's benefit, but rather to benefit others. Indeed, it may be very much against the patient's interests if, as it has been suggested, it inhibits the patient's right to a peaceful and dignified end.

The Law Commission left open the possibility that the question could be addressed in legislation (Law Commission, (v)). Should consensus be reached on this issue one option is for a person who is willing to have his/her organs used for transplantation and to be electively ventilated, to express this through some form of advance declaration. This could take the form of a donor card similar to the existing organ donor card, but perhaps in a different colour or shape to avoid confusion. It remains to be seen whether elective ventilation will receive sufficient public support to lead to legislative reform.

References

Andrews, K. *et al.* (1996) 'Misdiagnosis in a rehabilitative unit.' *BMJ*, **313**, 13.

BMA (1995) *Advance Statements About Medical Treatment.* BMA, London, (i) para 7.4; (ii) para 6.7; (iii) page 22.

BMA/RCN (1993) *Statement on Cardiopulmonary Resuscitation*. BMA/RCN, London.

Brazier, M. (1992) *Medicine, Patients and the Law*, 2nd edn. Penguin, Harmondsworth, (i) p. 274.

Dworkin, R. (1993) *Life's Dominion: An Argument About Euthanasia and Abortion.* Harper Collins, London.

Fletcher, N., Holt, J., Brazier, M. and Harris, J. *Nursing Law and Ethics.* Manchester University Press, Manchester, p. 210.

Fox, M. and McHale, J. (1997) 'Regulating xenotransplantation.' *NLJ*, **147**, 115.

House of Lords Select Committee on Medical Ethics (1994) HL Paper 21-I, HMSO, London.

Kennedy and Grubb (1994) *Evidence to the House of Lords Select Committee on Euthanasia Report* 31 January 1994.

Keown, J. (1991) Euthanasia in the Netherlands. *LQR*, 108, 51.

Law Commission (1995) *Mental Incapacity*. Law Commission No. 231, (i) para 5.30; (ii) para 5.34; (iii) 5.24; (iv) para 7.1; (v) 6.23–6.26.

Mason, J.K. (1990) 'Organ transplantation.' In *Doctors, Patients and the Law* (ed. C. Dyer). Blackwell Scientific, Oxford.

McHale, J.V. (1995) 'Elective ventilation – some ethical and legal problems.' *Professional Negligence*, 23.

New, B., Solomon, R., Dingwall, M. and McHale, J.V. (1994) *A Question of Give and Take*, Research Report No. 18. Kings Fund Institute, London.

RCN (1992) Living wills guidance for nurses. March; Ord. No. 00102, in the series *Issues in Nursing and Health.*

RCP (1996) *Criteria for the Diagnosis of Brain Stem Death – Review by a Working Group Convened by the Royal College of Physicians. Endorsed by the Conference of Medical Royal Colleges and their Faculties.* UK, RCP, London.

Schutz, S.E. (1994) 'Patient Involvement in Resuscitation Decisions.' *British Journal of Nursing*, **3**(20), 1075.

Skegg, P.D.K. (1984) *Law, Ethics and Medicine*, OUP, Oxford.

Stone, J. (1995) 'Withholding of life sustaining treatment.' *NLJ*, **145**, 354.

UKCC (1996) *Guidelines for Professional Practice*. United Kingdom Central Council for Nursing, Midwifery and Health Visiting, London, (i) para 32.

Wells, C. *et al.* (1990) 'An unsuitable case for treatment.' *NCJ*, 1544.

Appendix 1

Guidelines for professional practice

United Kingdom Central Council for Nursing, Midwifery and Health Visiting

Contents

Preamble

The UKCC has produced this booklet to provide a guide for reflection on the statements within the Code of Professional Conduct. For students and those of you who are new to the professions, we hope that you find it useful; others of you may be very familiar with the guidance provided. This booklet has been produced to help reflect on the many challenges that face us in day-to-day practice. This booklet should read as a whole and care should be taken to use each section in the context of all the guidance provided. It is important that time is taken to read and consider the whole document. You may find yourself in a crisis when there is no opportunity to reach for a book. At these times, you may need the guidance offered to make the professional judgement needed for that specific situation.

Once you have read the booklet, you will be able to dip into the relevant sections and we hope that you will use it regularly and reflect on the many subjects covered. Throughout this booklet, many general ethical and legal issues have been covered. However, it is important that you get to know the specific circumstances, safeguards, policies and procedures needed to provide treatment or care relevant to your area of practice.

The development of these guidelines has been a consultative process with input from individuals with different employment, education, consumer and practice backgrounds. It has been produced in order to replace and update the information provided in the following three documents; Exercising Accountability (March 1989), Confidentiality (April 1987) and Advertising by Registered Nurses, Midwives and Health Visitors (March 1985).

With the many challenges facing nurses, midwives and health visitors and the speed in which practice changes, we acknowledge that these guidelines for professional practice will require regular review. We will formally review the contents by June 1998 and, in the meantime, would welcome any comments you have. These should be sent to the Professional Officer, Ethics, at the UKCC's address.

Introduction

1 The UKCC's responsibilities are set out in the Nurses, Midwives and Health Visitors Acts for 1979 and 1992 and our main responsibility is to protect the interests of the public. To do this, we set standards for education, training and professional conduct for registered nurses, midwives and health visitors (registered practitioners). The motto on our coat of arms - 'care, protect, honour' - reflects these responsibilities. We hope that this booklet will help you to:
   - 'care' in a way that reflects your code of professional conduct (the UKCC Code of Professional Conduct 1992);
   - 'protect' patients and clients and
   - 'honour' your responsibilities as a registered practitioner.

2 With so many codes and charters about, it is easy to be confused about how they relate to your professional and personal life. The Code of Professional Conduct was drawn up by the UKCC under the powers of the Nurses, Midwives and Health Visitors Act 1979 to give advice to registered practitioners. This code sets out:
   - the value of registered practitioners;
   - your responsibilities to represent and protect the interests of patients and clients and
   - what is expected of you.

3 The role of the UKCC in protecting the public is firstly to maintain a register of people who are recommended to be suitable practitioners and who have demonstrated knowledge and skill through a qualification registered with the UKCC. Secondly, we can remove people from that register either because they are seriously ill or because a charge of misconduct has been proven against them. The code is used as the standard against which complaints are considered.

4 This booklet gives guidance on all sixteen clauses of the code. It deals with areas such as consent, truthfulness, advocacy and autonomy. It cannot deal with every conflict which a registered practitioner may face. We recognise that professional practice and decision-making are not straightforward. The circumstances we work under are always changing. The way we work must be sensitive and relevant and must meet the needs of patients and clients. We must be able to adjust our practice to changing circumstances, taking into consideration local procedures, policies and cultural differences.

Accountability - answering for your actions

5 As a registered practitioner, you hold a position of responsibility and other people rely on you. You are professionally accountable to the UKCC, as well as having a contractual accountability to your employer and accountability to the law for your actions. The Code of Professional Conduct sets our your professional accountability - to whom you must answer and how. The code begins with the statement that:

> "Each registered nurse,midwife and health visitor shall act, at all times, in such a manor as to: safeguard and promote the interests of individual patients and clients; serve the interests of society; justify public trust and confidence and uphold and enhance the good standing and reputation of the professionals."

Each clause of the code begins with the statement that:

> "As a registered nurse, midwife or health visitor, you are personally accountable for your practice and, in the exercise of your professional accountability, must..."

No one else can answer for you and it is no defence to say that you were acting on someone else's orders.

6 In exercising your profession accountability, there may be conflict between the interests of a patient or client, the health or social care team and society. This is especially so if health care resources are limited. Whatever decisions you take and judgements you make, you must be able to justify your actions.

7 Accountability is an integral part of professional practice, as in the course of practice you have to make judgements in a wide variety of circumstances. Professional accountability is fundamentally concerned with weighing up the interests of patients and clients in complex situations, using professional knowledge, judgement and skills to make a decision and enabling you to account for the decision made. Neither the Code of Professional Conduct nor this booklet seeks to state the circumstances in which accountability has to be exercised, but instead they provide principles to aid your decision making.

8 If you delegate work to someone who is not registered with the UKCC, your accountability is to make sure that the person who does the work is able to do it and that appropriate levels of supervision or support are in place.

9 The first four clauses of the code make sure that you put the interests of patients, clients and the public before your own interests and those of your professional colleagues. They are as follows:

> "As a registered nurse, midwife or health visitor, you are personally accountable for your practice and, in the exercise of your professional accountability, must...
> 1 act always in such a manner as to promote and safeguard the interests and well-being of patients and clients;
> 2 ensure that no action or omission on your part, or within your sphere of responsibility, is detrimental to the interests, condition or safety of patients and clients;
> 3 maintain and improve your professional knowledge and competence;
> 4 acknowledge any limitations in your knowledge and competence and decline any duties or responsibilities unless able to perform them in a safe and skilled manner;"

10 The code does not cover the specific circumstances in which you make decisions and judgements. It presents important themes and principles which you must apply to all areas of your work.

Duty of care

11 You have both a legal and a professional duty to care for patients and clients. In law, the courts could find a registered practitioner negligent if a person suffers harm because he or she failed to care for them properly. Professionally, the UKCC's Professional Conduct Committee could find a registered practitioner guilty of misconduct and remove them from the register if he or she failed to care properly for a patient or client, even though they suffered no harm.

12 Lord Atkin defined the duty of care when he gave judgement in the case of Donoghue v Stephenson (House of Lords) (1932). He said that:

> "You must take reasonable care to avoid acts or omission which you can reasonably foresee would be likely to injure your neighbour. Who, then, in the law is my neighbour? The answer seems to be persons who are so closely and directly affected by my act that I ought to have them in contemplation as being so affected when I am directing my mind to the acts or omissions which are called in question."

How circumstances can affect your duty of care

13 If there is a complaint against you, the UKCC's Professional Conduct Committee and possibly the courts would decide whether you took proper care. When they do this, they must consider whether what you did was reasonable in all the circumstances.

14 The following examples show how the duty of care changes according to the circumstances. Each example shows a skilled adult intensive care nurse in a different situation.

Example 1

The nurse is on duty in the intensive care unit when a patient suffers a cardiac arrest.

Here, it is reasonable to expect the nurse to care for the patient as competently as any experienced intensive care unit nurse.

Example 2

The nurse is walking along a hospital corridor and finds a women completely alone giving birth.

In this situation, it is not reasonable to expect the nurse to care for the women as a midwife would. But it is reasonable to expect the nurse to call a midwife or obstetrician and to stay with the women until appropriate help arrives.

Example 3

The nurse is walking along a street and comes across a person injured in a road traffic accident.

In this situation, the nurse does not have a legal duty to stop and care for the injured person. But if she does, she then takes on a legal duty to care for the person properly. In these circumstances, it is reasonable to expect her to care for the person to the best of her skill and knowledge. Although the nurse has no legal duty to stop and give care in this example, she does have a professional duty. The Code of Professional Conduct places a professional duty upon her at all times. However, in this situation it could be reasonable to expect the nurse to do no more than comfort and support the injured person.

What is reasonable?

15 The courts and the Professional Conduct Committee must decide whether your actions were reasonable. The case of Bolam v Friern Hospital Management Committee (1957) produced this test of what is reasonable:

> "The test is the standard of the ordinary skilled man exercising and professing to have that special skill. A man need not posses the highest expert skill at the risk of being found negligent ... it is sufficient if he exercises the skill of an ordinary competent man exercising that particular art."

16 This test is usually called the Bolam test. Although the case concerned a doctor, the Bolam test can be used to examine the actions of any professional person. The case of Wilsher v Essex AHA (1988) set the standard of reasonable care to be expected of students and junior staff. The standard is that of a reasonably competent practitioner and not that of a student or junior. You have a duty to ensure that the care which you delegate is carried out at a reasonably competent standard. This means that you remain accountable for the delegation of the work and for ensuring that the person who does the work is able to do it. The Code of Professional Conduct provides principles which you can apply to any situation. If you use these principles, you will be able to carry out your legal and professional duty of care.

Withdrawing care to protect the public and yourself

17 There may be circumstances of conflict where the registered practitioner may consider withdrawing his or her care. A situation like this might occur if the registered practitioner fears physical violence or if there are health and safety hazards involved in providing care. There may be other situations where the registered practitioner may seek support or consider withdrawing care, for example due to sexual or racial harassment. Any decision to withdraw care has to be taken very carefully and you should first discuss, if possible, the matter with managers, the patient's or client's family and, if appropriate and wherever possible, the patient or client themselves. In certain circumstances, you may need help to make sure that the public are safe. If possible, you should discuss this with other members of the health care team. However, in areas of practice where violence may occur more frequently, such as in some areas of mental health care and in accident and emergency departments, there must be protocols to deal with these situations. Appropriate training and on-call support arrangements should also be available. In all cases, you should make a record of the fact that you withdrew care so that if your actions or decisions are questioned, you can justify them.

Patient and client advocacy and autonomy

18 Recognising a patient's or client's right to choose is clearly outlined in clauses 1 and 5 of the code. Although the words advocacy and autonomy are not specifically used, it is this section which states the registered practitioner's role in these respects. The code states that:

> "As a registered nurse, midwife or health visitor, you are personally accountable for your practice and, in the exercise of your professional accountability, must...
> 1 ...act always in such a manner as to promote and safeguard the interests and well-being of patients and clients; (advocacy) ...
> 5 ...work in an open and co-operative manner with patients, clients and their families, foster their independence and recognise and respect their involvement in the planning and delivery of care;" (autonomy)

19 The registered practitioner must not practise in a way which assumes that only they know what is best for the patient or client, as this can only create a dependence and interfere with the patient's or client's right to choose. Advocacy is concerned with promoting and protecting the interests of patients or clients, many of whom may be vulnerable and incapable of protecting their own interests and who may be without the support of family or friends. You can do this by providing information and making the patient or client feel confident that he or she can make their own decisions. Advocacy also involves providing support if the patient refuses treatment/care or withdraws their consent. Other health care professionals, families, legal advisors, voluntary agencies and advocates appointed by the courts may also be involved in safeguarding the interests of patients and clients.

20 Respect for patients' and clients' autonomy means that you should respect the choices they make concerning their own lives. Clause 5 of the code outlines your professional role in promoting patient/client independence. This means discussing with them any proposed treatment or care so that they can decide whether to refuse or accept that treatment or care. This information should enable the patient or client to decide what is in their own best interests.

21 Registered practitioners must respect patients' and clients' rights to take part in decisions about their care. You must use your professional judgement, often in conjunction with colleagues, to decide when a patient or client is capable of making an informed decision about his or her treatment and care. If possible, the patient or client should be able to make a choice about his or her care, even if this means that they may refuse care. You must make sure that all decisions are based on relevant knowledge. The patient's or client's right to agree to or refuse treatment and care may change in law depending on their age and health. Particular attention to the legal

position of children must be given, as their right to give consent or refuse treatment or care varies in different parts of the United Kingdom and depending on their age.

Communicating

22 Communication is an essential part of good practice. The patient or client can only make an informed choice if he or she is given clear information at every stage of care. You also need to listen to the patient or client. Listening is a vital part of communication. Effective communication relies on all our skills. Building a trusting relationship will greatly improve care and help to reduce anxiety and stress for patients and clients, their families and their carers. For effective communication, you may need to consult other colleagues with specialist knowledge, or you may need the services of interpreters to make sure that information is understood. It is important to create an environment for good communication so that you can build a relationship of trust with the patient or client. Employers should recognise the importance of communication when they plan staffing structures and levels.

23 To ensure that you gain the trust of your patients and clients, you should recognise them as equal partners, use language that is familiar to them and make sure that they understand the information you are giving. Your records must also be clear, legible and accessible to the patient or client, as outlined in the UKCC's document Standards for Records and Record Keeping and under the terms of the Data Protection Act 1984 and the Access to Health Records Act 1990. Written communication is as important as verbal communication.

Truthfulness

24 Patients and clients have a legal right to information about their condition; registered practitioners providing care have a professional duty to provide such information. A patient or client who wants information is entitled to an honest answer. There may be rare occasions when a person's condition and the likely effect of information given at a specific time might lead you to be selective (although never untruthful) about the information you give. Any decision you make about what information to give must be in the best interests of the patient or client.

25 There is potential for disagreement or even conflict between different professionals and relatives over giving information to a patient

or client. When discussing these matters with colleagues or relatives, you must stress that your personal accountability is firstly to the patient and client. Any patient or client can feel relatively powerless when they do not have full knowledge about their care or treatment. Giving patients and clients information helps to empower them. For this reason, the importance of telling the truth cannot be overestimated. If patients or clients do not want to know the truth, it should not be forced upon them. You must be sensitive to their needs and must make sure that your communication is effective. The patient or client must be given a choice in the matter. To deny them that choice is to deny their rights and so diminish their dignity and independence.

Consent

26 You must obtain consent before you can give any treatment or care. The patient's or client's decision whether or not to agree to treatment must be based on adequate information so that they can make up their mind. It is important that this information is shared freely with the patient or client, in an accessible way and in appropriate circumstances. In emergency situations, where treatment is necessary to preserve life and the patient or client cannot make a decision (for example because they are unconscious), the law allows you to provide treatment without the patient's or client's consent, always acting in the best interests of the patient or client. You should also know that if the patient or client is an adult, consent from relatives is not sufficient on its own to protect you in the event of challenge, as nobody has the right to give consent on behalf of another adult.

27 When the patient or client is told about proposed treatment and care, it is important that you give the information in a sensitive and understandable way and that you give the patient or client enough time to consider it and ask questions if they wish. It is not safe to assume that the patient or client has enough knowledge, even about basic treatment, for them to make an informed choice without an explanation. You must respect the patient's or client's decision, regardless of whether he or she agrees to or refuses treatment.

28 It is essential that you give the patient or client adequate information so that he or she can make a meaningful decision. If a patient or client feels that the information they received was insufficient, they could make a complaint to the UKCC or take legal action. Most legal action is in the form of an allegation of negligence. In exceptional cases, for example where a patient's or client's consent was obtained by deception or where not enough information was given, this could result in an allegation of battery (or civil assault in Scotland). However, only in the most extreme cases is criminal law likely to be involved.

Who should obtain consent?

29 It is important that the person proposing to perform a procedure should obtain consent, although there may be some urgent situations where another practitioner can do so. Sometimes you may not be responsible for obtaining a patient's or client's consent as, although you are caring for the patient or client, you would not actually be carrying out the procedure. However, you are often best placed to know about the emotions, concerns and views of the patient or client and may be best able to judge what information is needed so that it is understood. With this in mind, you should tell other members of the health care team if you are concerned about the patient's or client's understanding of the procedure or treatment, for example, due to language difficulties.

Types of consent

30 Although the most important aspect of obtaining consent is providing and sharing information, the patient or client may demonstrate their decision in a number of ways. If they agree to treatment and care, they may do so verbally, in writing or by implying (by co-operating) that they agree. Equally a patient or client may withdraw or refuse consent in the same way. Verbal consent, or consent by implication, will be enough evidence in most cases. You should obtain written consent if the treatment or care is risky, lengthy or complex. This written consent stands as a record that discussions have taken place and of the patients's or client's choice. If a patient or client refuses treatment, making a written record of this is just as important. You should make sure that a summary of the discussions and decisions is placed in the patient's or client's records.

When consent is refused

31 Legally, a competent adult patient can either give or refuse consent to treatment, even if that refusal will shorten their life. Therefore you must respect the patient's refusal just as much as you would their consent. You must make sure that the patient is fully informed and, when necessary, involve other members of the health care team. As before, you should make sure that a summary of the discussions is placed in the patient's or client's records.

32 Increasingly, the law and professional bodies are also recognising the power of advanced directives or living wills. These are documents made in advance of a particular condition arising and they show the patient's or client's treatment choices, including the decision not to accept further treatment in certain circumstances. Although not necessarily legally binding, they can provide very useful information

about the wishes of a patient or client who is now unable to make a decision and therefore should be respected.

Consent of people under 16

33 If the patient or client is under the age of 16 (a minor), you must be aware of local protocols and legislation that affect their care or treatment. Consent of patients or clients under 16 is very complex, so you may need to seek local, legal or membership organisation advice. Some of the laws relating to a minor's consent have been referenced at the back of this booklet.

Consent of people who are mentally incapacitated

34 It is important that the principles governing consent are applied just as vigorously to all forms of care with people who are mentally incapacitated as with a competent adult. A patient or client may be described as mentally incapacitated for a member of reasons. There may be temporary reasons such as sedatory medicines or longer term reasons such as mental illness, coma or unconsciousness.

35 When a patient or client is considered incapable of providing consent, or where the wishes of a mentally incapacitated patient or client appear to be contrary to the interests of that person, you should be involved in assessing their care or treatment. You should consult relevant people close to the patient or client, but respect any previous instructions the patient or client gave.

36 In some cases of legal incapacity, such as when a patient is in a persistent vegetative state, certain decisions will need court authority. Court authority may also be necessary or desirable in decisions concerning selective non-treatment of handicapped infants, dealing with certain circumstances of neonate care or sterilisation of a mentally handicapped individual.

Mental Health Acts

37 If you are involved in the care or treatment of patients or clients detained under statutory powers in the Mental Health Acts, you must get to know the circumstances and safeguards needed for providing treatment and care without consent.

Making concerns known

38 Employers have a duty to provide the resources needed for patient and client care, but the numerous requests to the UKCC for advice on this subject indicate that the environment in which care is provided

is not always adequate. You may find yourself unable to provide good care because of a lack of adequate resources. Also, you may be afraid to speak out for fear of losing your job. However, if you do not report your concerns, you may be in breach of the Code of Professional Conduct. You may also have concerns over inappropriate behaviour by a colleague and feel it necessary to make your concerns known. You will need to report your concerns to the appropriate person or authority, depending on the type of concerns. You may feel it necessary to discuss these decisions with other colleagues or a membership organisation.

39 The clauses of the code which relate specifically to these issues are numbers 11, 12 and 13:

> "As a registered nurse, midwife and health visitor, you are personally accountable for your practice and, in the exercise of your professional accountability, must ...
>
> 11 report to an appropriate person or authority, having regard to the physical , psychological and social effects on patients and clients, any circumstances in the environment of care which could jeopardise standards of practice;
>
> 12 report to an appropriate person or authority any circumstances in which safe and appropriate care for patients and clients cannot be provided;
>
> 13 report to an appropriate person or authority where it appears that the health and safety of colleagues is at risk, as such circumstances may compromise standards of practice and care;"

40 These clauses give advice on the minimum action to be taken. This will help to make sure that those who manage resources and staff have all the information they need to provide an adequate and appropriate standard of care. You must not be deterred from reporting your concerns, even if you believe that resources are not available or that no action will be taken. You should make your report verbally and/or in writing and,where available, follow local procedures. The manager (who may also be registered with us) should assess the report and communicate it to senior managers where appropriate. This is important because if, subsequently, any complaint is made about the registered practitioners involved in providing care, this may require senior managers to justify their actions if inadequate resources are seen to affect the situation.

41 As outlined in clauses 11, 12 and 13 of the code, the registered practitioner's role is to make sure that safe and appropriate care is provided. This means:

- promoting staff support throughout care settings;
- telling senior colleagues about unacceptable standards;
- supporting and advising colleagues at risk;

- reporting circumstances in the environment which could jeopardise standards of practice;
- making sure that local procedures are in place, challenged and/or changed;
- being aware of new codes, charters and registration body guidelines;
- keeping accurate records and
- when necessary, obtaining guidance on how to present information to management.

Working together

42 The UKCC recognises the complexity of health care and stresses the need to appreciate the contribution of professional health care staff, students, supporting staff and also voluntary and independent agencies. Providing care is a multi-professional, multi-agency activity which, in order to be effective, must be based on mutual understanding , trust, respect and co-operation. Patients and clients are equal partners in their care and therefore have the right to be involved in the health care team's decisions.

43 Under clause 6 and clause 14 of the Code of Professional Conduct:

> "As a registered nurse, midwife or health visitor, you are personally accountable for your practice and, in the exercise of your professional accountability, must ...
>
> 6 work in a collaborative and co-operative manner with health care professionals and others involved in providing care, and recognise and respect their particular contributions within the care team;...
>
> 14 assist professional colleagues, in the context of your own knowledge, experience and sphere of responsibility, to develop their professional competence and assist others in the care team, including informal carers, to contribute safely to a degree appropriate to their roles;"

These clauses emphasise the importance of support and co-operation and also the importance of avoiding disputes and promoting good relationships and a spirit of co-operation and mutual respect within the health and social care team. It is clearly impossible for any one profession to possess all the knowledge, skills and resources needed to meet the total health care needs of society. Good care should be the product of a good team.

44 Good team work is important but co-operation and collaboration are not always easily achieved, for example, if:

- individual members of the team have their own specific and separate objectives or

- one member of the team tries to adopt a dominant role without considering the opinions, knowledge and skills of its other members.

In such circumstances, achieving good team work needs hard work and negotiation between all the health care professionals involved. In all the discussions, it is important to stress that the interests of the patient or client must come first.

45 Discrimination has no place in health care. This means making sure that equal opportunities policies are in place, challenged and/or changed and ensuring that no one has to endure racial or sexual harassment. Each member of a team is entitled to equality and must not be discriminated against because of gender, age, race, disability, sexuality, culture or religious beliefs. There needs to be effective communication and team work to make sure these principles are not neglected.

Conscientious objection

46 In today's developing health service, you may find yourself in situations which you find very uncomfortable. There may be many circumstances in which a practitioner, due to personal morality or religious beliefs, will not wish to be involved in a certain type of treatment or care. Clause 8 of the Code of Professional Conduct states that:

> "As a registered nurse, midwife or health visitor, you are personally accountable for your practice and, in the exercise of your professional accountability, must ...
>
> 8 report to an appropriate person or authority, at the earliest possible time, any conscientious objection which may be relevant to your professional practice;"

47 In law, you have the right to conscientiously to object to take part in care in only two areas. These are the Abortion Act 1967 (Scotland, England and Wales), which gives you the right to refuse to take part in an abortion, and the Human Fertilisation and Embryology Act 1990, which gives you the right to refuse to participate in technological procedures to achieve conception and pregnancy.

48 However, in an emergency, you would be expected to provide care. You should carefully consider whether or not to accept employment in an area which carries out treatment or procedures to which you object. If, however, a situation arises in which you do not want to take part in a form of treatment or care, then it is important that you declare your objection in time for managers to make alternative arrangements. In certain circumstances, this may mean providing counselling for the staff involved in these decisions. You do not have the right to refuse to take part in emergency treatment.

49 Refusing to be involved in the care of patients because of their condition or behaviour is unacceptable. The UKCC expects all registered practitioners to be non-judgmental when providing care. This is one of the issues addressed by clause 7 of the code, which states that:

> "As a registered nurse, midwife or health visitor, you are personally accountable for your practice and, in the exercise of your professional accountability, must ...
> 7 recognise and respect the uniqueness and dignity of each patient and client, and respect their need for care, irrespective of their ethnic origin, religious beliefs, personal attributes, the nature of their health problems or any other factor;"

Confidentiality

50 To trust another person with private and personal information about yourself is a significant matter. If the person to whom that information is given is a nurse, midwife or health visitor, the patient or client has a right to believe that this information, given in confidence, will only be used for the purposes for which it was given and will not be released to other without their permission. The death of a patient or client does not give you the right to break confidentiality.

51 Clause 10 of the Code of Professional Conduct addresses this subject directly. It states that:

> "As a registered nurse, midwife or health visitor, you are personally accountable for your practice and, in the exercise of your professional accountability, must ...
> 10 protect all confidential information concerning patients and clients obtained in the course of professional practice and make disclosures only with consent, where required by the order of a court or where you can justify disclosure in the wider public interest;"

Confidentiality should only be broken in exceptional circumstances and should only occur after careful consideration that you can justify your action.

52 It is impractical to obtain the consent of the patient or client every time you need to share information with other health professionals or other staff involved in the health care of that patient or client. What is important is that the patient or client understands that some information may be made available to others involved in the delivery of their care. However, the patient or client must know who the information will be shared with.

53 Patients and clients have a right to know the standards of confidentiality maintained by those providing their care and these standards

should be made known by the health professional at the first point of contact. These standards of confidentiality can be reinforced by leaflets and posters where the health care is being delivered.

Providing information

54 You always need to obtain the explicit consent of a patient or client before you disclose specific information and you must make sure that the patient or client can make an informed response as to whether that information can be disclosed.

55 Disclosure of information occurs:
- with the consent of the patient or client;
- without the consent of the patient or client when the disclosure is required by law or by order of a court and
- without the consent of the patient or client when the disclosure is considered to be necessary in the public interest.

56 The public interest means the interests of an individual, or groups of individuals or of society as a whole, and would, for example, cover matters such as serious crime, child abuse, drug trafficking or other activities which place others at serious risk.

57 There is no statutory right to confidentiality but an aggrieved individual can sue through a civil court alleging that confidentiality was broken.

58 The situation that causes most problems is when your decision to withhold confidential information or give it to a third party has serious consequences. The information may have been given to you in the strictest confidence by a patient or client or by a colleague. You could also discover the information in the course of your work.

59 You may sometimes be under pressure to release information but you must realise that you will be held accountable for this. In all cases where you deliberately release information in what you believe to be the best interests of the public, your decision must be justified. In some circumstances, such as accident and emergency admissions where the police are involved, it may be appropriate to involve senior staff if you do not feel that you are able to deal with the situation alone.

60 The above circumstances can be particularly stressful, especially if vulnerable groups are concerned, as releasing information may mean that a third party becomes involved, as in the case of children or those with learning difficulties.

61 You should always discuss the matter fully with other professional colleagues and, if appropriate, consult the UKCC or a membership organisation before making a decision to release information without a patient's permission. There will often be significant consequences which you must consider carefully before you make a decision, you should write down the reasons either in the appropriate record or in

a special note that can be kept in a separate file (outlined in the UKCC's booklet Standards for Records and Record Keeping). You then have written justification for the action which you took if this becomes necessary and you can also review the decision later in the light of future developments.

Ownership of and access to records

62 Organisations which employ professional staff who make records are the legal owners of these records, but that does not give anyone in that organisation the legal right of access to the information in those records. However, the patient or client can ask to see their records, whether they are written down or on computer. This is as a result of the Data Protection Act 1984, Access Modification (Health) Order 1987 and the Access to Health Records Act 1990.

63 The contracts of employment of all employees not directly involved with patients but who have access to or handle confidential records should contain clauses which emphasise the principles of confidentiality and state the disciplinary action which could result if these principles are not met.

64 As far as computer-held records are concerned, you must be satisfied that as far as possible, the methods you use for recording information are secure. You must also find out which categories of staff have access to records to which they are expected to contribute important personal and confidential information. Local procedures must include ways of checking whether a record is authentic when there is no written signature. All records must clearly indicate the identity of the person who made that record. As more patient and client records are moved and linked between health care settings by computer, you will have to be vigilant in order to make sure that patient or client confidentiality is not broken. This means trying to ensure that the systems used are protected from inappropriate access within your direct area of practice, for example ensuring that personal access codes are kept secure.

65 The Computer Misuse Act 1990 came into force to secure computer programs and data against unauthorised access or alteration. Authorised users have permission to use certain programs and data. If those users go beyond what is permitted, this is a criminal offence. The Act makes provision for accidentally exceeding your permission and covers fraud, extortion and blackmail.

66 Where access to information contained on a computer filing system is available to members of staff who are not registered practitioners, or health professionals governed by similar ethical principles, an important clause concerning confidentiality should appear within their contracts of employment (outlined in the UKCC's position statement Confidentiality: use of computers, 1994).

67 Those who receive confidential information from a patient or client should advise them that the information will be given to the registered practitioner involved in their care. If necessary, this may also include other professional in the health and social work fields. Registered practitioners must make sure that, where possible, the storage and movement of records within the health care setting does not put the confidentiality of patient information at risk.

Access to records for teaching, research and audit

68 If patients' or clients' records need to be used to help students gain the knowledge and skills which they require, the same principles of confidentiality apply to the information. This also applies to those engaged in research and audit. The manager of the health care setting is responsible for the security of the information contained in these records and for making sure that access to the information is closely supervised. The person providing the training will be responsible for making sure that students understand the need for confidentiality and the need to follow local procedures for handling and storing records. The patient or client should know about the individual having access to their records and should be able to refuse that access if they wish.

69 In summary, the following principles concerning confidentiality apply:

- a patient or client has the right to expect that information given in confidence will be used only for the purpose for which it was given and will not be released without their permission;
- you should recognise each patient's or client's right to have information about themselves kept secure and private;
- if it is appropriate to share information gained in the course of your work with other health or social work practitioners, you must make sure that as far as is reasonable, the information will be kept in strict professional confidence and be used only for the purpose for which the information was given;
- you are responsible for any decision which you make to release confidential information because you think that this is in the public's best interest;
- if you choose to break confidentiality because you believe that this is in the public's best interest, you must have considered the situation carefully enough to justify that decision and
- you should not deliberately break confidentiality other than in exceptional circumstances.

Advertising and sponsorship

70 Clause 16 of the UKCC's Code of Professional Conduct addresses the subject of the promotion of commercial goods or services. It states that:

"As a registered nurse, midwife or health visitor, you are personally accountable for your practice and, in the exercise of your professional accountability, must...

16 ensure that your registration status is not used in the promotion of commercial products or services, declare any financial or other interests in relevant organisations providing such goods or services and ensure that your professional judgement is not influenced by any commercial considerations."

71 Patients or clients and their relatives or friends are often anxious when attending hospitals and other health care facilities. The environment of care should help to promote good health, healing and recovery and not be one of commercial advertising.

72 Clause 16 does not intend to prevent registered practitioners employed in positions such as the matron of a private nursing home or as a representative of a pharmaceutical company, or who are offering their professional services privately, from using their registration status on items such as business cards and headed note paper.

73 However, if a practitioner has a direct financial or other direct interest in an organisation providing commercial goods or services, for example, a ward sister who is discharging a patient to a nursing home owned and run by herself or one of her relatives, then that practitioner must make her interests known.

74 It is also unacceptable for registered practitioners to carry commercial advertising or promotional material on their uniforms.

75 Under the Code of Professional Conduct, registered practitioners must protect the interests of patients and clients, be worthy of public trust and confidence and avoid using professional qualifications in ways which might compromise the independence of professional judgements upon which patients and clients rely. The vulnerability of patients and clients is reflected by these elements of the code, which also indicate the importance of trust between a registered practitioner and a patient as well as the expectation that the registered practitioner will respond to the patient's need unconditionally.

Sponsorship

76 Funding for some posts, projects or services is sometimes offered by companies, some of which have a commercial interest in matters associated with health care. Sponsorship arrangements which affect the professional judgement of registered practitioners and patient or client choice should be bought to the attention of those who provide health care services.

77 Students on pre-registration and post-registration courses often need sponsorship to carry out their study, especially for overseas study visits. The decision to accept sponsorship must be made by the individual, taking account of the appropriateness of the support offered.

Receiving gifts

78 You may be offered gifts, favours or hospitality from patients or clients during the course of or after a period of care or treatment. The Code of Professional Conduct states that:

> "As a registered nurse, midwife and health visitor, you are personally accountable for your practice and, in the exercise of your professional accountability must ...
> 15 refuse any gift, favour or hospitality from patients or clients currently in your care which might be interpreted as seeking to exert influence to obtain preferential consideration;"

The important principles is not that the registered practitioner never receives gifts or favours but that they could never be interpreted as being given by the patient or client in return for preferential treatment.

Complementary and alternative therapies

79 Complementary therapies are gaining popularity and finding a more substantial place in health care. It is vitally important that you ensure that the introduction of any of these therapies to your practice is always in the best interests and safety of the patients and clients. Clause 9 of the code outlines your privileged relationship with patients and clients:

> "As a registered nurse, midwife and health visitor, you are personally accountable for your practice and, in the exercise of your professional accountability must ...
> 9 avoid any abuse of your privileged relationship with patients and clients and of the privileged access allowed to their person, property, residence or workplace;"

The registered practitioner therefore must be convinced of the relevance and accountability of the therapy being used and must be able to justify using it in a particular circumstance, especially when using the therapy as part of professional practice. It should also be part of professional team work to discuss the use of complementary therapies with medical and other members of the health care team caring for the particular patient or client.

80 Some registered practitioners, who successfully complete courses in complementary or alternative therapies not usually associated with their professional practice, quote their registration status when advertising their services. The UKCC believes that a person's registration status should not be needed to support a complementary or alternative therapy course or qualification if the course is valid and credible. However, if it is a registered practitioner's registered status that gives

credibility to the qualification, then the registered practitioner must use their own judgement and discretion to make sure that they are not misleading the public.

81 If a complaint is made against you, we can call you to account for any activities carried out outside conventional practice. You should carefully consider the content and status of any courses which you undertake and how you promote yourself.

Research and audit

82 Increasing numbers of registered practitioners are carrying out, or are involved in, research or audit. The results might improve practice, help to audit an aspect of clinical services, inform policy or be part of a graduate or postgraduate qualification. Other practitioners are employed or involved with clinical trials which force on new treatments, new technology or improvements to patient care.

83 If you are involved in these activities, issues often arise which you need to consider. Is the research ethical? Is your role appropriate? Has the Local Research Ethics Committee (LREC) given its approval? Has local management given their approval? What is the make-up of the LREC? Are there registered practitioners on the LREC?

Types of research

84 The range of research carried out varies greatly. Outlined below are some of the types of research that are used in the health care setting.

Projects

85 An increasing number of students are being asked to do project work for diplomas or undergraduate degrees. Many educational institutions recommend that their diploma or undergraduate students do not become involved in clinically-based research.

86 As the number of these projects increases, contact with patients or clients might be refused. This is quite reasonable, as the care and comfort of patients or clients must always be considered. Projects by registered practitioners may be promoted by developments at clinical level, by involvement in practice units or as a result of participating in clinical supervision.

Higher degrees

87 Research for postgraduate degrees is supervised and guided throughout. It is important to gain approval for research in clinical areas from

management in addition to consulting the local LREC before starting the work.

Other research work and clinical research trials

88 Research activities intended to benefit patient care or investigate practice are carried out by a wide range of clinicians, academics and others. Registered practitioners may be involved in this work as part of their job, because of academic interest or in response to a perceived or expressed need.

89 Contracts of employment specify how practitioners must work. They do not always cover concerns about the ethics of research, confidentiality, consent or other issues. Under European Community Directive 91/507/EEC, all elements of clinical trials carried out within the European Union must adhere to the guidelines on good clinical practice for trials on medical protocols in the EU. These guidelines provide a useful framework for nurses, midwives and health visitors to use when they are involved in research work.

90 If there is contact with patients or clients, it is important for you to discuss the benefits of the work with the appropriate manager. You must be certain that approval from the LREC is obtained. Repeated requests for patients and clients to fill in questionnaires or to be interviewed can be intrusive and potentially disruptive to care. For this reason, the views of patients, clients, and their associates will assist in determining prospective compliance.

Criteria for safe and ethical conduct of research

91 You must always refer to the UKCC's Code of Professional Conduct and The Scope of Professional Practice. These documents provide the framework for all actions of registered nurses, midwives and health visitors.

92 As well as using these documents, you need to be sure that the research or clinical trial you are carrying out meets specific criteria. These are that:

- the project must be approved by the LREC;
- management approval must be gained where necessary;
- arrangements for obtaining consent must be clearly understood by all those involved;
- confidentiality must be maintained;
- patients must not be exposed to unacceptable risks;
- patients should be included in the development of proposed projects where appropriate;
- accurate records must be kept and
- research questions need to be well structured and aimed at producing clearly anticipated care or service outcomes and benefits;

93 You need to consider these criteria before submitting a research proposal to a LREC. You are expected to participate fully in the design process and this includes raising legitimate concerns when they arise. If no LREC exists in your area, it is important to refer to local policy for research.

Audit

94 Audit seeks to improve practice and treatment and to reduce risk by the systematic review of the process and outcome of care and treatment and by the evaluation of records and other data. There are occasions when contact with patients and clients, carers or relatives is necessary and therefore LREC clearance may be required. Consideration of the other points highlighted above is recommended.

Conclusion

95 We have produced this booklet to help you in your professional practice. It would be impossible to discuss all the issues faced by registered practitioners. Answers are not always straightforward. The Code of Professional Conduct and The Scope of Professional Practice apply to all registered practitioners and the interests of the public, patients and clients are of the greatest importance. You should also remember that being accountable and working with those who provide care is the foundation upon which the best standards are achieved. With the many challenges facing nurses, midwives and health visitors and the speed in which practice changes, it is acknowledged that these guidelines for professional practice will require regular review. We will formally review these guidelines by June 1998 and, in the meantime, would welcome any comments which you may have. Comments on this booklet should be sent to the Professional Officer, Ethics, at the UKCC's address.

96 In producing this booklet, we have been greatly helped by comments from representatives of practice, education, medical, professional, membership and consumer organisations. We have tried to produce the booklet in a form that is easily accessible in order to aid professional judgement and to outline basic principles.

97 If you need further information or advice, please contact our team of professional officers at the:

Standards Promotion Directorate
United Kingdom Central Council
for Nursing, Midwifery and Health Visiting
23 Portland Place
London W1N 4JT
Telephone: 0171 637 7181
Fax: 0171 436 2924

Documents relevant to these guidelines

1 *Code of Professional Conduct*, UKCC, 1992
2 *The scope of Professional Practice*, UKCC, 1992
3 *Midwives Rules*, UKCC, 1993
4 *The Midwife's Code of Practice*, UKCC, 1994
5 *Standards for Records and Record Keeping*, UKCC, 1993
6 *Standards for the Administration of Medicines*, UKCC, 1992
7 *Confidentiality: use of computers, position statement*, UKCC, 1992
8 *Complementary therapies, position statement*, UKCC, 1995
9 *Acquired Immune Deficiency Syndrome and Human Immune Deficiency Virus Infection (AIDS and HIV infection)*, UKCC, 1994
10 *Anonymous Testing for the Prevalence of the Human Immune Deficiency Virus (HIV)*, UKCC, 1994

These documents are available on written request from the Distribution Department at the UKCC.

Laws relevant to these guidelines

1 Nurses, Midwives and Health Visitors Acts 1979 and 1993
2 Access to Health Records Act 1990
3 Family Law Reform Act 1969
4 Age of Legal Capacity (Scotland) Act 1991
5 Children Act 1989
6 Mental Health (Northern Ireland) Order 1986
7 Mental Health (England and Wales) Act 1983
8 Mental Health (Scotland) Act 1984
9 Abortion Act 1967
10 Human Fertilisation and Embryology Act 1990
11 Data Protection Act 1984
12 Access Modification (Health) Order 1987
13 Computer Misuse Act 1990
14 European Community Directive 91/507/EEC

These are available from your local branch of Her Majesty's Stationery Office (HMSO).

Appendix 2

The Health Service Ombudsman

England

1. General guidance

The Health Service Ombudsman investigates complaints about the National Health Service (NHS). Before asking the Ombudsman to look into your complaint, you must first take it up locally with your local hospital, clinic or surgery. **Section 2** tells you what to do first.

If you are not happy with the way your complaint has been dealt with locally, write to the Ombudsman giving all the details. You do not need to employ a lawyer to put your complaint to the Ombudsman. There is a detachable form in the middle of this leaflet which you can use if you wish.

Section 5 tells you what kinds of complaints the Ombudsman can investigate. There are some complaints which the Ombudsman *cannot* take up and **Section 6** tells you what they are. It is not possible in this leaflet to deal with every possibility. If you are not sure whether the Ombudsman can help, you can write or telephone for advice. The address and telephone number are at the back of this leaflet.

Section 7 explains what happens when the Ombudsman receives your complaint.

The Ombudsman is **completely independent** of the NHS and the Government. There is **no charge** for the Ombudsman's service.

This leaflet is currently available in Welsh, large print, tape, symbol summary and in the following languages: Arabic, Bengali, Chinese, Greek, Gujerati,

Hindi, Punjabi, Urdu, Somali, Sinhalese, Turkish and Vietnamese.

2. How to make your complaint

The first steps – local investigation

You need first to take up your complaint locally. Your hospital, clinic or surgery can tell you how to do that. You can ask them for a leaflet which will have the details. Most complaints can be settled quickly in this way – by letter or by discussion with you.

If you are not satisfied after that, you can ask the local NHS Trust or Health Authority for a review of your complaint by an independent panel. If your request is granted, the review will be carried out by a panel usually of three members. The panel will be chaired by an independent person.

Involving the Ombudsman

The Ombudsman will not normally become involved unless you have used **both** these local stages and are still unhappy, for example, because:

- it took too long to deal with your complaint locally;
- you were unreasonably refused a panel review;
- you did not get a completely satisfactory answer to your complaint.

Who can complain to the Ombudsman?

The person complaining can be:-

- the patient
- a relative (normally the closest member of the family)
- someone else, for example someone who works for the NHS or a Community Health Council.

If you complain on behalf of a patient, you must explain why the patient is not doing so. You must also say whether the patient supports the complaint.

Time limits

You have to send your complaint to the Ombudsman no later than a year from the date when you became aware of the events which are the subject of complaint. The Ombudsman can sometimes extend the time limit, but only if there are special reasons. One reason might be that the local investigation of your complaint took much longer than it should have done.

3. Putting your complaint to the Ombudsman

You should write and:

- describe what happened, when, where and (if you can) who was involved;
- say why you are complaining. You need to show that there has already been hardship or injustice. The Ombudsman does not investigate something that might cause problems in the future;
- provide all the evidence you can. Send all your letters and any background papers. If you send originals, photocopies will be taken (at no cost to you) and the originals returned to you promptly;
- if you can, please include a telephone number where you can be contacted during the day.

You can use the form with this leaflet or just write a letter. The form tells you what information the Ombudsman will need to know.

Before you write, please look at:

- Section 5 – which tells you what the Ombudsman *can* investigate
- Section 6 – which tells you what the Ombudsman *cannot* investigate.

4. Getting help

Your local Community Health Council will be able to help you. Otherwise you can ask for help from a Citizens Advice Bureau or from your Member of Parliament.

Telephone numbers and addresses for your local Community Health Council, Citizens Advice Bureau and Member of Parliament are in the phone book, available in your local library.

5. What can the Ombudsman investigate?

The Ombudsman can investigate complaints about hospitals or community health services which are about:

a. a poor service;
b. failure to purchase or provide a service you are entitled to receive;
c. maladministration – that is administrative failures such as:

- avoidable delay
- not following proper procedures
- rudeness or discourtesy
- not explaining decisions
- not answering your complaint fully and promptly.

Where the matters you are complaining about happened after 31 March 1996, the Ombudsman may also investigate:

d. complaints about the care and treatment provided by a doctor, nurse or other trained professional;
e. other complaints about family doctors (GPs), or about dentists, pharmacists or opticians providing a NHS service locally.

Complaints about access to information

You have rights to information about how the NHS operates locally. These are set out in the Government's Code of Practice on Openness in the NHS. Copies of the Code should be available in your local library or from your local hospital. If you ask your Health Authority or Trust for information and are not content with the response you first receive, you should write to the chief executive of the Health Authority or NHS Trust concerned. If you remain dissatisfied you can complain to the Ombudsman about such things as:

- refusal to provide the information – unless it is something you do not have the right to see;
- a delay of over four weeks in getting the information requested;
- the level of any charge you are asked to pay for it.

Such information may be about the services available locally, the standards set or achieved, or the details of important decisions or proposals.

Under the Code you can also ask for information about the NHS services provided by your local general practitioner, dentist, pharmacist or optician. If you are not satisfied with the reply you receive you may complain to the Ombudsman.

Please note

The Ombudsman does not have to investigate your complaint. **It is up to the Ombudsman to decide whether to take up any particular complaint**. If your complaint is not to be investigated, you will be told why.

6. Matters that the Ombudsman cannot investigate

The Ombudsman cannot look into:

a. complaints which you could take to **court** or **an independent tribunal** – unless the Ombudsman does not think it reasonable for you to do so. If you are seeking damages for what has happened, only the courts can decide that. The Ombudsman cannot take up your complaint at all if you have already started legal action;

b. **personnel issues** such as appointments of staff, pay or discipline. The Ombudsman cannot investigate complaints from NHS staff about their employment. The Ombudsman **can** look into complaints from staff about the way in which a complaint about them by or on behalf of a patient has been handled by a NHS Authority or Trust;

c. **commercial or contractual matters**, unless they relate to services for patients provided under a NHS contract;

d. **properly made decisions** a NHS authority or other body or individual providing NHS services has a right to make even if you do not agree with the decision;

e. **services in a non-NHS hospital or nursing home**, *unless* they are paid for by the NHS;

f. complaints about **government departments**, such as

the Department of Health or the NHS Executive. Those complaints are for the Parliamentary Ombudsman to consider;

g. complaints about **local authority** departments, such as social services. Those complaints are for the Local Government Ombudsman to consider.

7. How will the Ombudsman deal with your complaint?

First stage

When your complaint is received by the Ombudsman, a decision will be made on whether or not an investigation will be carried out. If the Ombudsman cannot look into your complaint or decides not to, you will be told why.

Investigation

If the Ombudsman decides to investigate, you will be sent a statement of complaint. It will set out for you and for the body to be investigated what matters the Ombudsman will look into. The body which is responsible for the matters to be investigated will be asked to send to the Ombudsman their comments and all relevant papers – which might include your medical records (these will be kept strictly confidential).

After those papers have been received and studied a member of the Ombudsman's staff may ask to interview you at a convenient time and place. You can have a friend of your choice with you. The Ombudsman's investigator may then interview others concerned. If your complaint is about treatment provided by doctors, nurses or other professionals, independent professional advisers will be available to help the Ombudsman with the investigation.

Interviews are carried out in private. They are usually informal, although the Ombudsman has the same power as the civil courts to obtain evidence. Because the Ombudsman's investigations are thorough, they can take several months.

The report

At the end of the investigation you will be sent the Ombudsman's report. A copy is also sent to the NHS or other body responsible for the matters you complained about. If your complaint is found to be justified, the Ombudsman will seek for you an apology or other remedy. Sometimes that may include getting a decision changed, or a repayment of unnecessary costs to patients or their families. The Ombudsman does not recommend damages. The Ombudsman may also call for changes to be made so that what has gone wrong does not happen again. Where the body you complained about tells the Ombudsman that it will make such changes, the Ombudsman checks that they have done so.

Is there any appeal against the Ombudsman's decisions?

No. A complaint to the Ombudsman is the final stage in the procedure for pursuing a complaint. The Ombudsman's decision on a complaint is final. If completely new information comes to light which could reasonably have been known about before, the Ombudsman may start a new investigation. That is extremely rare.

THE HEALTH SERVICE OMBUDSMAN'S ADDRESS AND TELEPHONE NUMBER ARE:

The Health Service Ombudsman for England
Millbank Tower
Millbank
London SW1P 4QP
Telephone 0171 217 4051
Text telephone 0171 217 4066

Before you post your letter, or the form with this leaflet, have you

- said what your complaint is?
- said who is involved?
- said when, and where, what you are complaining about happened?
- enclosed all the correspondence with the NHS or other body locally to whom you have complained, including other papers about your complaint?
- given your address and, if possible, a daytime telephone number?

HEALTH SERVICE OMBUDSMAN COMPLAINT FORM

It will help the Ombudsman if you fill in the form as far as you can. Section four of the leaflet tells you how to get help if you need it.

Please read the leaflet carefully before you decide to make a complaint. The leaflet tells you what the Ombudsman can and cannot investigate.

Please use block capitals when answering questions 1 to 6. Where you are given a choice of YES/NO, circle the **correct** answer.

ABOUT YOU

1. Name ______________________

2. Address ______________________

____

____

______________ Postcode ______________

3. Daytime telephone number

____

4. Are you the patient involved in the complaint? YES NO

If the answer is yes, please go to question 12

ABOUT THE PATIENT

5. Name ______________________

6. Address ______________________

____

____

______________ Postcode ______________

7. What is your relationship to the patient?

____

____

8. Has the patient died? YES NO

If the answer is no, please go to question 10

9. Are you the next of kin? YES NO

If not, does the next of kin support your approach to the Ombudsman? YES NO

Please read the note at the end of this form before answering this question

Please go to question 12

10. Please explain why the patient cannot make the complaint

____

____

____

____

____

11. Does the patient know that you are making a complaint and support it? YES NO

Please read the note at the end of this form before answering this question

ABOUT THE BODY (OR BODIES) YOU ARE COMPLAINING ABOUT

12. Which NHS body(ies) or other body are you complaining about?

____

____

____

____

13. Please give the name and, if possible, the job title of the person you complained to at the body concerned.

____

____

____

____

14. Was your complaint made in writing? YES NO

15. Have you received a reply? YES NO

ABOUT YOUR COMPLAINT

If you have more than one complaint, if possible, please complete questions 16 - 21 separately for each complaint. Please continue on a separate sheet of paper if necessary.

16. What are you complaining about?

____

____

____

____

Please continue on reverse

HEALTH SERVICE OMBUDSMAN COMPLAINT FORM

17. How have you or the patient been affected?

18. What has the body you complained to done about it?

19. Why are you not satisfied with what it has done?

20. What do you want the Ombudsman to find out or do for you?

21. On what date did you first know of the matter(s) you are complaining about? If it is more than one year ago, please explain why you did not complain to the Ombudsman sooner.

PAPERS TO SUPPORT YOUR COMPLAINT

22. Before the Ombudsman can consider a complaint, all the papers need to be seen, particularly letters to and from the body you are complaining about. All originals will be returned after copying.

Are you sending the Ombudsman all the papers?
YES NO

If not, please say, if possible, which papers you cannot provide.

23. The Ombudsman may, if necessary and with your permission, decide to obtain papers you do not send from the NHS body. Do you agree to this?
YES NO

LEGAL ACTION? (See section 6 of the leaflet).

24. Are you planning legal action? YES NO

Name
(IN BLOCK CAPITALS) ______

Signed ______

Date ______

Please send this form, and any background papers, to the following address:

Office of the Health Service Ombudsman
Millbank Tower, Millbank
London SW1P 4QP

Note on questions 9 and 11
In question 9 the Ombudsman needs to know if the next of kin supports the complaint because the next of kin may be interviewed in any investigation. The Ombudsman will not normally investigate if the next of kin does not support the complaint. For the same reason the Ombudsman needs to know, in question 11, whether the patient supports the complaint. The Ombudsman will not normally investigate if the patient does not support the complaint.

Appendix 3

Complaints procedures

Local resolution for trusts/health authorities

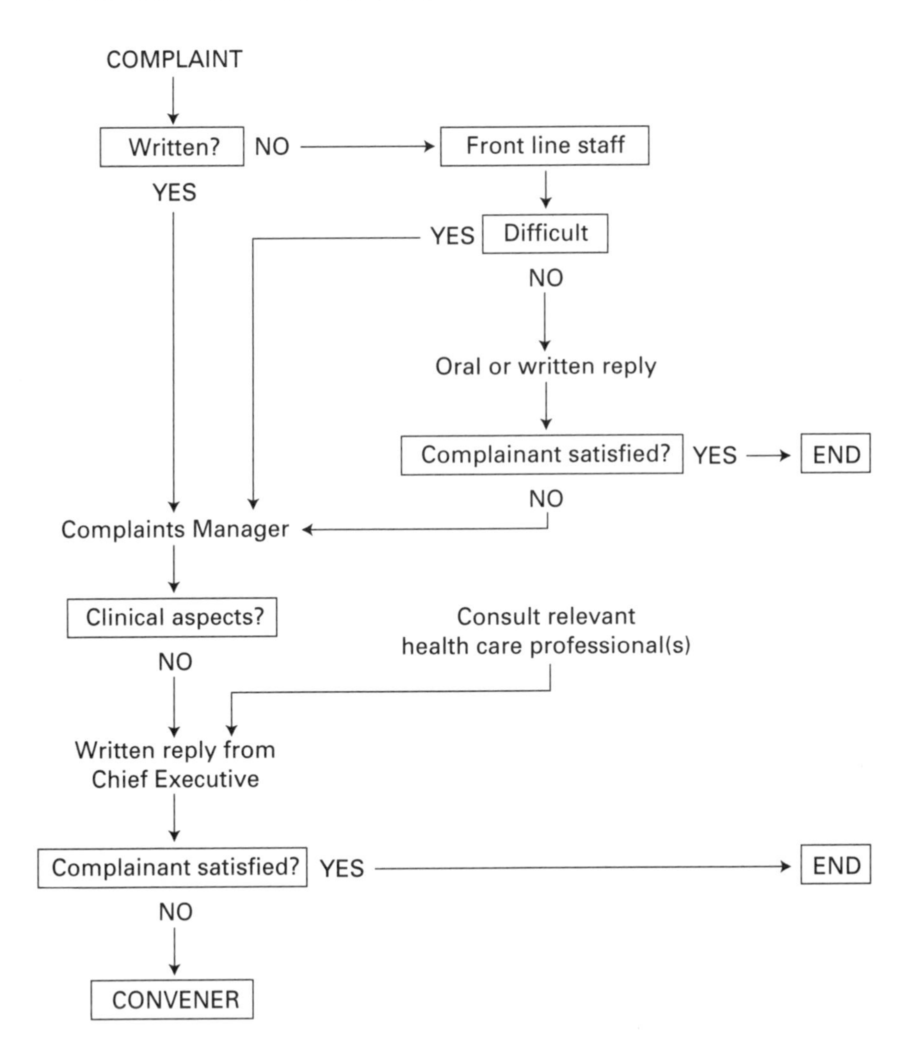

Independent review for trusts and health authorities

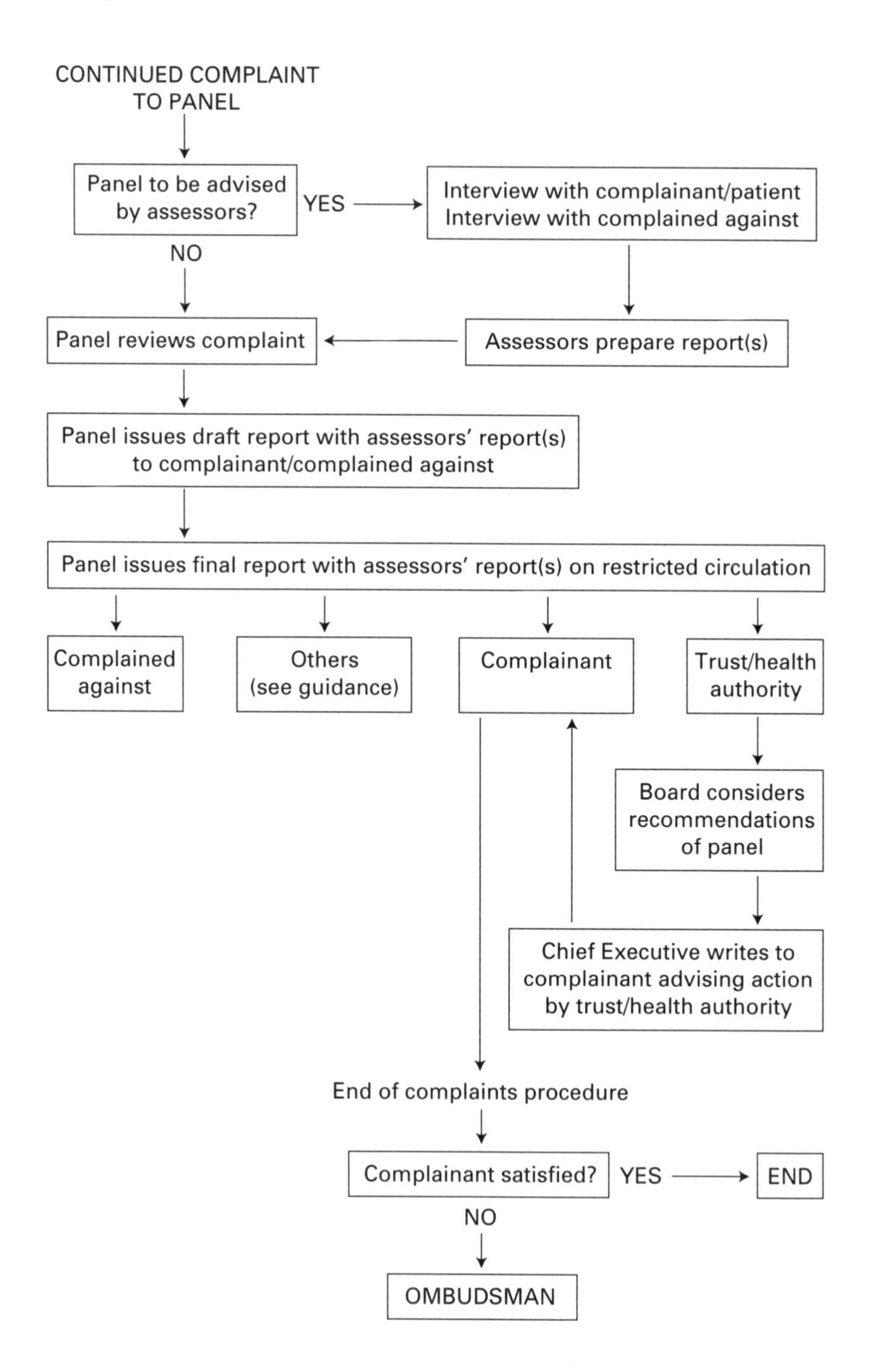

Independent review for family health services practitioners

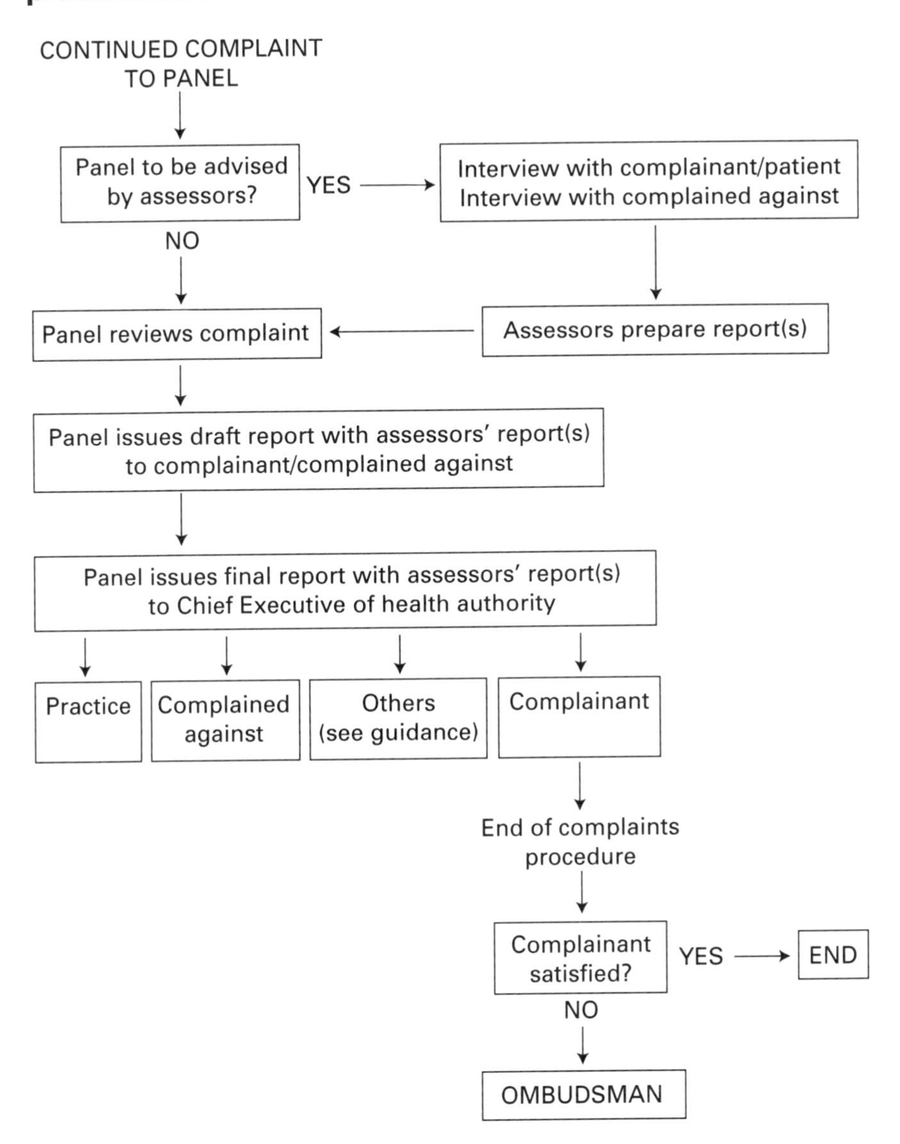

Index